COMMON FACTORS
IN COUPLE AND FAMILY THERAPY

Common Factors in Couple and Family Therapy

The Overlooked Foundation for Effective Practice

Douglas H. Sprenkle
Sean D. Davis
Jay L. Lebow

THE GUILFORD PRESS
New York   London

© 2009 The Guilford Press
A Division of Guilford Publications, Inc.
370 Seventh Avenue, Suite 1200, New York, NY 10001
www.guilford.com

Paperback edition 2014

Printed in the United States of America

This book is printed on acid-free paper.

Last digit is print number: 9   8   7   6

Library of Congress Cataloging-in-Publication Data

Sprenkle, Douglas H.
   Common factors in couple and family therapy : the overlooked foundation
for effective practice / Douglas H. Sprenkle, Sean D. Davis, Jay L. Lebow.
      p. cm.
   Includes bibliographical references and index.
   ISBN 978-1-60623-325-2 (hardcover : alk. paper)
   ISBN 978-1-4625-1453-3 (paperback : alk. paper)
   1. Couples therapy.   2. Family psychotherapy.   3. Marital psychotherapy.
I. Davis, Sean D.   II. Lebow, Jay.   III. Title.
   RC488.5.S725 2009
   616.89′1562—dc22
                                                                    2009019250

About the Authors

Douglas H. Sprenkle, PhD, until his death in 2018, was Professor Emeritus at Purdue University, where he was developer and former Director of the Doctoral Program in Marriage and Family Therapy. Dr. Sprenkle was past Editor of the *Journal of Marital and Family Therapy* and the author or editor of over 130 scholarly articles and books. He received the Osborne Award from the National Council on Family Relations, which is given biannually for outstanding teaching, and the Outstanding Contribution to Marriage and Family Therapy Award, the Cumulative Career Contribution to Marriage and Family Therapy Research Award, and the Training Award from the American Association for Marriage and Family Therapy. Dr. Sprenkle also won the Award for Significant Contribution to Family Therapy Theory and Practice from the American Family Therapy Academy.

Sean D. Davis, PhD, is Associate Professor at the Couple and Family Therapy Program at Alliant International University's campus in Sacramento, California, as well as an approved supervisor and clinical member of the AAMFT. Dr. Davis also serves on the editorial board of the *Journal of Marital and Family Therapy*. His research, clinical, and teaching interests focus on common factors and bridging the scientist–practitioner gap in marriage and family therapy. His dissertation on common factors won the 2005 AAMFT Graduate Student Research Award and the 2006 AAMFT Dissertation Award. Dr. Davis has published several journal articles and books, including, most recently, *What Makes Couples Therapy Work?* and *The Family Therapy Treatment Planner, Second Edition* (with Frank M. Dattilio and Arthur Jongsma), and maintains a private practice.

Jay L. Lebow, PhD, is Clinical Professor of Psychology at the Family Institute at Northwestern University. He has conducted clinical practice, supervision, and research on couple and family therapy for over 30 years. He is board certified in family psychology by the American Board of Professional Psychology and is an approved supervisor of the AAMFT. Dr. Lebow is the author of 100 book chapters and articles, most of which focus on the interface of research and practice and the practice of integrative couple and family therapy. His published books include *Research for the Psychotherapist* and four edited volumes, including the *Handbook of Clinical Family Therapy*. He is a past president of the Division of Family Psychology of the American Psychological Association and is involved in the Family Institute's Psychotherapy Change Project. Dr. Lebow is the current editor of *Family Process*.

Acknowledgments

All three of us would like to acknowledge the common factors intellectual giants on whose shoulders we have stood in writing this book, including but not limited to Carl Rogers, Saul Rosenzweig, Jerome Frank, Michael Lambert, Bruce Wampold, and the decades of psychotherapy research on common factors carried out by members of the Society for Psychotherapy Research. We also wish to thank Jim Nageotte of The Guilford Press for the special attention he gave to this project.

I (D. H. S.) would like to extend a special word of thanks to Barry Duncan, Scott Miller, and Mark Hubble, who first encouraged me to write in this area in their pioneering volume *The Heart and Soul of Change*. I also want to acknowledge the significant input of Adrian Blow, my friend and frequent collaborator in my common factors publications. I also want to give thanks to my students and colleagues in the Doctoral Program in Marriage and Family Therapy at Purdue University who have listened to these ideas and challenged them for the past decade. The "Purdue Mafia" will always hold a special place in my heart. To my coauthors, Sean Davis and Jay Lebow, I thank you for writing chapters that only you could have written and for contributing to the exciting synergy in this volume. It was an honor to work with you! Finally, major appreciation is reserved for my spouse, Sidney Moon, who has championed my work for decades, been a indefatigable listening ear, and loved me more than I have ever deserved.

I (S. D. D) would like to thank my early mentors in the field, particularly Drs. Mark Butler, Fred Piercy, and Doug Sprenkle. You are each truly consummate professionals; in addition to having a lengthy list of professional accomplishments, each of you is humble, unpretentious, and kind. Much of what is good in my professional and personal life is a result of our friendships. Doug Sprenkle and Jay Lebow, you have been a delight to work with; your collegial spirit and passion for common factors have made the daunting task of writing a book fun. I would also like to thank my colleagues and students at Alliant International University—our ongoing dialogues have forced me to refine and clarify my ideas on the conceptualization and application of common factors. Most important, I thank my wife, Elizabeth. Without your tireless support, my participation in this book would still be a dream. I never cease to be amazed by you. To my children, Andrew, Hannah, Rachel, and William, thank you for insisting that I step away from my projects and attend to your skinned knees, take you to the park, and jump with you on the trampoline. Being your dad has taught me more about being therapeutic than anything I have learned in my profession. And yes, the book is done and your dad is back!

I (J. L. L.) would like to thank my mentors, Ken Howard and David Orlinsky, for instilling an understanding of the importance of common factors and generic principles of psychotherapeutic change in the formative years in my career; this foundation has served me well even in the context of the multitasking required in couple and family therapy. I also would like to thank my colleague Bill Pinsof, whose work on alliance and therapy progress has been a continual inspiration in our collaboration over many years and whose pioneering efforts revealed ways common factors apply to a systemic context. Most especially, I would like to thank my colleagues Doug Sprenkle and Sean Davis for being so thoughtful, patient, and delightful in our long-distance collaboration.

Contents

COMMON FACTORS
IN COUPLE AND FAMILY THERAPY

1

What Is Responsible for Therapeutic Change?

Two Paradigms

W*hat is responsible for therapeutic change?* Science offers many examples of misguided assumptions about causality. Until the early 1980s, the majority of physicians as well as lay people believed peptic ulcers were caused by worry, stress, and personality variables (or by excessive coffee drinking or spicy foods). Today we know that about 90% of peptic ulcers are primarily caused by the *H. pylori* bacteria, which typically can be treated successfully through a 1- to 2-week regimen of antibiotics.

When I (D. H. S.) was growing up, most people thought "good foods" were those rich in vitamins. I was encouraged to eat a lot of spinach since it was high in vitamins A and C. I was discouraged from eating blueberries since they had few vitamins and therefore did not contain the essential ingredients that caused good health. Now we know that phytochemicals make a much greater contribution to wellness and that some foods like blueberries, with relatively few vitamins, are loaded with phytochemicals that powerfully promote health. In this instance, while vitamins contribute to good health, they turned out to be not as central as science had previously assumed.

This book challenges the commonly held assumption that what causes change in psychotherapy is primarily the unique ingredients in therapy models and techniques. While, like vitamins, these ingredients are typically beneficial and we hold them in high regard, we nonetheless challenge their centrality in the process of change. We also think that the question "What is responsible for therapeutic change?" should be incredibly important to the psychotherapeutic practitioner, as well as to the theoretician and the researcher. For the answer surely guides what we do in the consulting room, determines how we view or explain what we do, and should be the focus of what we investigate.

Our answer to this question differs from how we (the three authors of this book) were trained and goes against the grain of most of the most powerful forces in the psychotherapy establishment. This book sets forth an emerging paradigm (common-factors-driven change) of why therapy works, with a special emphasis on how this paradigm plays out in couple and family therapy. In brief, this paradigm suggests that psychotherapy works predominantly not because of the unique contributions of any particular model of therapy or unique set of interventions (what we call the model-driven change paradigm) but rather because of a set of common factors or mechanisms of change that cuts across all effective therapies. We further believe that this emerging view has powerful implications for therapists, supervisors, and trainers, and that mastering this approach will improve your results.

As is discussed in more detail in the next chapter, while we call it "emerging," this paradigm is not technically "new." Its roots go back over 70 years, and there has been a vocal minority of scholars and clinicians within psychotherapy that has long advocated for it (Karasu, 1986; Lambert, 1992; Lambert & Ogles, 2004; Luborsky, Singer, & Luborsky, 1975). There has also been a small group of relationship therapists (Hubble, Duncan, & Miller, 1999) upon whose ideas we have built the particulars of our approach. But the paradigm remains "emerging" in the sense that it remains a countercultural minority position that is not consciously at the center of the practice of most psychotherapists or important to the major funding agencies like the National Institutes of Health (NIH) or the psychotherapy research establishment. These groups largely remain committed to the model-driven paradigm.

The three authors of this book are all practicing therapists (with a special emphasis in couple and family therapy). Although we also teach and do research at universities, we see individuals, couples, and families on a daily basis and have the hearts of clinicians. Because we work in the trenches, we will endeavor to speak to practitioners as the primary audience for this book. We also, however, share a lifelong passion for thinking about why change occurs, and we believe that theory-driven (as opposed to "seat-of-the-pants") therapy is likely to be more coherent and effective. Hence, we try to engage you, the reader, in the theoretical rationale for our approach under the assumption that there is "nothing as practical as a good theory." Finally, we are also applied researchers who value evidence. We came to believe in this emerging paradigm because we thought the evidence for it is more compelling than for the earlier paradigm. Wherever possible, then, we do not expect you simply to take our word for these ideas but instead offer data that we think support the emerging paradigm. In sum, this book is written for practitioners and students who are open to being theoretically and research-informed.

Two Paradigms of Therapeutic Change

If you ask most psychotherapists why change occurs, they would explain the process primarily in terms of their preferred model of change. A structural family therapist, for example, might say that change occurs when the therapist facilitates families' changing their organizational pattern—like from rigid or diffuse boundaries to clear boundaries. A narrative therapist might say that change occurs when therapists encourage clients to reauthor their lives from disempowering, subjugated life stories to self-narratives that are empowering and self-efficacious. Common factors that cut across all successful therapies might be mentioned and might even be valued (considered necessary), but they would not likely be considered the major reasons that change occurs. Instead, the emphasis would be on the unique contribution of the model.

If you had asked all three of us the same question 10–15 years ago, we probably would have probably answered it in terms of the earlier paradigm. For me (D. H. S.), it would have never occurred to me to think otherwise. Remember that a paradigm is a large interpretive framework that shapes how we see things, and until and unless we undergo a paradigm shift, it is almost impossible for us to view things differently. When I came into the couple and family therapy field in the 1970s, it was the "golden age" of the great model developers, and I remember being mesmerized at workshops by such luminaries as Salvador Minuchin, Carl Whitaker, Virginia Satir, Jay Haley, and James Framo. What these people seemed to be doing with clients was so remarkable that I never questioned that what was responsible for therapeutic change was anything other than the specific contributions of each model. For me, the only real question was which models were "true" and which model or models should guide my work.

Couple and family therapy, of course, is not unique in its fascination with models. At least 400 different models of psychotherapy have been documented as model developers have continued the unending quest to answer the question that opened this chapter. Indeed, this proliferation of models led Sol Garfield (1987) to quip, "I am inclined to predict that sometime in the next century there will be one form of psychotherapy for every adult in the Western world" (p. 98). One potential benefit, then, of adopting the new paradigm is that it may no longer be necessary to continue inventing new models (Sprenkle & Blow, 2004a)!

Some of the major factors that distinguish the two paradigms—old and new—are depicted in Figure 1.1. In the explanations that follow the figure, we make clear that the two paradigms are not polar opposites but rather represent matters of emphasis that probably exist along a continuum. We also believe that there is some merit to the model-driven change paradigm. We will elaborate on these ideas in Chapter 5 when we talk about our "moderate" approach to common factors.

More details of the two paradigms will be supplied in later chapters. In keeping with our thesis that the two paradigms are not

Model-driven change	**Common-factors-driven change**
Primary Explanation for Change	
Emphasizes the unique elements and mechanisms of change within each model.	Emphasizes the common mechanisms of change that cut across all effective psychotherapies; models are the vehicles through which common factors operate.
Guiding Metaphor	
Medical: considers treatment as analogous to medical procedures and drugs.	*Contextual*: believes such qualities as credibility, alliance, and allegiance "surrounding" the treatment are more important than the unique aspects of treatment.
Therapists' Role in Change	
Emphasizes the treatment that is dispensed rather than who offers it.	Asserts that the qualities and capabilities of the person offering the treatment are more important than the treatment itself.

(continued)

Clients' Role in Change

More therapist-centric: although therapy can be collaborative, places greater emphasis on the value of the therapist's performing the treatment in a *specified manner*; and invests a stronger conviction in clients using the treatment in the ways the therapist intends and recommends.	More client-centric: places less importance on performing the treatment in a specific way and more on improvising to match the clients' needs and world views; and invests a stronger conviction in clients using whatever is offered in therapy for their own purposes in often unique and idiosyncratic ways.

Place in the Culture

Most funded research (e.g., NIH research) emphasizes this paradigm; represents the majority voice; and advocates lists of "approved" treatments.	Funding sources deemphasize this paradigm; represents the minority voice; and opposes lists of "approved" treatments.

FIGURE 1.1. Two paradigms of therapeutic change.

opposite entities, we underscore the observation that models *do* play an important role in common-factors-driven change. However, proponents of our favored paradigm see models less as unique sources of change than the vehicles through which common factors operate. Therapists need models to give their work coherence and direction, but this paradigm values them more for their capacity to activate common mechanisms of change found in all successful psychotherapies.

The older model uses a medical lens through which to view psychotherapy—hardly surprising, given that the earliest psychotherapists were physicians. It follows that many psychotherapy researchers believe that therapies "are analogous to medications that need to be assessed in tightly controlled research that establishes specific variants of therapy as safe and effective for the treatment of particular disorders; essentially drug research without the drugs" (Lebow, 2006b, p. 31). In his well-documented challenge to the medical model, Wampold (2001) makes a strong empirical case for the greater impact of certain "contextual" qualities that surround treatment—like "allegiance" (the commitment of the therapist to the model) and "alliance" (the quality of the client–therapist relationship and the extent to which clients believe therapists are on the "same page"); and he documents empirically that a number of other variables *not* specific to the treatment contribute more to the outcome variance in psychotherapy than the "specific" treatment factors do.

Of course, we think that the medical model has done wonders for medicine. We also believe it has been very beneficial for psychotherapy to the extent that it has encouraged the use of randomized clinical trials in psychotherapy research to demonstrate that psychotherapy "works." Because of these trials we can say to external audiences, like third-party payers, with considerable confidence that psychotherapy (both individual and relational) is very effective (Wampold, 2001; Shadish & Baldwin, 2002). We will never understate the importance of this hard-fought knowledge gained through clinical trials research.

However, it is one thing to say that we know that psychotherapy is effective but quite another to say that we know *why* psychotherapy is effective. While appreciating the contributions of the medical model, we argue against the medical model assumptions that the various "treatments" explain the "why" and that comparative treatments should be the primary focus of research attention in the same way that competing drugs are the focus in drug investigations.

Another major difference between the two paradigms is the role of the therapist. It follows, in the older paradigm, that if psychotherapies are like medications, then the treatment being "dispensed" is much more important than who administers it. As Lebow (2006) has put it:

> Psychotherapy researchers typically focus exclusively on different clinical interventions while ignoring the psychotherapists who make use of them. It's as if treatment methods were like pills, in no way affected by the person administering them. Too often researchers regard the skills, personality, and experiences of the therapist as side issues, features to control or to ensure that different treatment groups receive comparable interventions. (pp. 131–132)

In the emerging paradigm, the role of the therapist is essential to activating the model or treatment, and without the therapist's expertise the model is little more than words on a piece of paper. New-paradigm advocates suggest that the role of the therapist is underemphasized in traditional psychotherapy research, given its emphasis on pitting treatments against one another. This focus also flies in the face of common sense since it is obvious that therapists differ in their effectiveness. As Wampold (2001) has noted, just as some lawyers achieve better outcomes than others, some artists produce more memorable sculptures, and some teachers engender greater student achievement, it only makes sense that some therapists will achieve better results. In spite of these truisms, the older paradigm gives relatively little attention to therapist variables as contributors to outcome. We present the empirical case for differences in therapist effectiveness in Chapter 4.

Because of its emphasis on the unique treatment being offered, the older paradigm often ends up being more therapist-centric. Granted, it would be inaccurate to say that all model-driven therapists see therapy as something they "do" as an "expert" to a relatively passive client. Many model-driven therapists, especially those with a social constructionist bent, work in ways that are very collaborative. Nonetheless, we believe there is often a tendency—*if* a therapist believes that change is due to a very specific set of operations found within a treatment model—to focus more on "dispensing" or "performing" those specific operations. And this "true believer" therapist will more likely believe that how faithfully he or she performs those specific operations will determine whether change occurs. When change does occur, we believe this therapist is also more likely to believe the client will think the change is due to these unique operations. In other words, this therapist will believe that the clients use the therapy in the way that the therapist thinks he or she uses it. For example, the structural family therapist will believe that the family in treatment was successful because its members used the therapy to develop more clear boundaries. Similarly, the narrative therapist will believe that therapy was successful because his or her clients learned to create new and more empowering stories about themselves.

In the newly emerging paradigm, there is more of a tendency to see clients as actively utilizing *whatever is offered for their own purposes*. While the family in treatment may have used the therapy to develop more clear boundaries, or to develop more empowering narratives, alternately family members may believe they have changed because they used the therapy to learn how to manage their differences or to gain insight about how to perform better at work (or any one of myriad other explanations that were not central to the therapist's belief as to why the treatment succeeded). Of course, both the therapist's and the clients' perspectives may be "valid," but the new paradigm privileges the clients' interpretation. Therapists who take the time to ask their clients why they think therapy succeeded are often shocked to discover that clients often say it had little to do with the therapists' cherished explanations (Helmeke & Sprenkle, 2000). Our central point here is that clients using whatever is offered for their own purposes largely explains or accounts for the robust finding (Shadish & Baldwin, 2002; Wampold, 2001) that there are typically only modest differences in the results achieved by very disparate therapies that independently have been shown to be effective. For example, in the largest and arguably the best psychotherapy outcome study ever completed, cognitive-behavioral therapy for depression achieved no better results than interpersonal therapy, a psychodynamic treatment (Elkin et al., 1989). Shadish and Baldwin (2002) have demonstrated that the results of 20 meta-analyses show no differences or only modest ones between the various seemingly disparate relational therapies. That is, clients use whatever is offered, in their own idiosyncratic ways, to achieve their goals.

I (D. H. S.), for example, have even had numerous experiences with clients totally misinterpreting me and later thanking me for something I never intended to say or do. For example, a recently divorced woman told me her life changed dramatically for the better when she became single; and she thanked me for "telling" her to leave her husband. I believe I bent over backwards to help her look at all sides of her ambivalence during divorce decision-making therapy and never "told" her what to do. If anything, I thought I encouraged hope for the relationship throughout couple and individual sessions with this client. She used—as clients often do—whatever the therapist offered for her own purposes in getting better.

Finally, engaging and motivating clients is at the heart of the new paradigm since the client's involvement is more important than the therapist's specific activity. In fairness, though, some old paradigm models give considerable attention (along a continuum from considerable to very little) to engaging and motivating clients, and so, once again, we don't want to portray the two paradigms as "either–or."

Finally, the old paradigm is much more entrenched in the dominant culture. Lebow (2006) points out that the medical model-type research "makes up the preponderance of research on mental health treatment funded over the last 20 years by the National Institutes of Health" (p. 31). It is much more closely aligned with the *Diagnostic and Statistical Manual of Mental Disorders* (DSM) power structure in that it assumes certain mental health "diagnoses" are best treated by manualized models demonstrated to be "effective" in randomized clinical trials. In fairness, however, the NIH does fund process research, and so it is not the case that its entire emphasis is on comparative treatment research. So, to repeat, the contrasts between the two paradigms should not be overdrawn. Proponents of the model-driven paradigm push for approved "lists" of efficacious treatments, and there is a growing trend in the mental health provider establishment to reimburse only for treatments put on these lists.

Although the new paradigm has a strong research base (Shadish & Baldwin, 2002; Wampold, 2001), most common factors research is not funded by major sources like NIH, since this type of research focuses not on unique treatments but, rather, shared sources of variance in therapeutic outcomes. While proponents see some value in the DSM as a way of reliably identifying patterns of symptoms, they reject the notion that a diagnosis alone is a meaningful basis for treatment planning since, for example, the etiology of "major depression" is too varied to prescribe limited treatment options. Furthermore, they believe the notion of "lists" of approved treatments is misguided since they reject, among other things, the notion that what makes treatments effective are their unique elements. They believe that this movement too readily embraces the most commonly researched models (typically cognitive behavior and its variations) when other approaches (often better suited to particular therapists) are likely to be just as effective. Given the varied and changing needs of clients, proponents of common factors also want to make a larger place for therapist *improvisation*. The proponents of the new paradigm are considered at least somewhat "countercultural" and at times are even labeled gadflies, iconoclasts, or rebels.

In summary, advocates of the two paradigms typically use the same ingredients, but they view them very differently. Just as the Ptolemaic and Copernican paradigms both included the earth, the sun, and the planets but saw their interrelationships differently, similarly advocates of both the old and the emerging paradigms of change use the same phenomena—models, therapists, clients, and the process of change—but see their interrelations differently. It is our contention (invoking Gregory Bateson's famous phrase) that it is a "difference that will make a difference" in your clinical work. For example, if your competence as a therapist—independent of the model you adopt—is more important than the model itself, you are likely to search for common ingredients in therapist expertise and push for researchers to learn more about these variables.

The Broad and Narrow Conceptualizations of Common Factors

Although our definition of "common factors" focuses on those variables that contribute to change that are not the province of any particular theoretical approach or model, we acknowledge that common factors can be narrowly and broadly defined. The narrow view (Lambert, 1992) conceptualizes them in terms of common aspects of interventions found in disparate models under different names (for example, creating changes in meaning may be labeled "insight," "reframing," or "externalizing the problem"). The broad conceptualization (Hubble et al., 1999) sees common factors as including other dimensions of the treatment setting—like client, therapist, relationship, and expectancy variables. From this perspective, for example, one can see "therapist variables" (characteristics of the therapist that contribute to the outcome) as a common factor since it is quite clear that therapist competence (independent of whatever model he or she employs) is an important contributor to outcome. Generally speaking, the broader approach is favored throughout this book. But whether broadly or narrowly defined, common factors can be contrasted with *specific* factors—those variables that contribute to outcome that are unique to a particular approach or model.

Resistance to Common Factors among Relational Therapists

We believe that there appears to be more resistance to the common factors paradigm among relational therapists than among individual therapists. This heightened resistance may be attributable to the fact that the application of common factors to couple and family therapy did not appear in the literature to any great extent prior to the 1990s. Nonetheless, we also believe that the history of relationship therapy has tended to emphasize differences—first, in order to differentiate it from mainstream psychotherapy and, second, from other relational approaches. Couple and family therapy model developers have typically been highly charismatic individuals with exceptional capacities to "sell" their models and gain adherents. This emphasis on distinctiveness was made easier because the field has not been particularly influenced by research but has grown more on the basis of intuitive or emotional appeal (Nichols & Schwartz, 2001). In addition, the field has historically focused on difficult cases, and this tendency may have contributed to the belief that unique models and methods are necessary for successful outcomes. Moreover, the field has always welcomed innovation and may therefore attract people with an above-average need to believe what they are doing is uniquely relevant. For whatever reasons, relationship therapists seem to be very emotionally invested in their models, and there may be simply too much cognitive dissonance for them to admit that their pet theories may not be demonstrably superior after all. Finally, since couple and family therapies are frequently promoted by charismatic figures on the workshop circuit, such an undramatic approach as common factors may seem dull by comparison. As Frank (1976) expressed it, "Little glory derives from showing that the particular method one has mastered with such effort may be indistinguishable from other methods in its effects" (p. 47). Of course, not all model developers are charismatic, and some value evidence more than dogma; but we maintain that the field has had more than its share of religion masquerading as science.

The Plan for This Book

Foundations of Common Factors in Couple and Family Therapy

The first five chapters are foundational and more general. Chapter 2 traces the history of common factors. While the contemporary history stretches back to 1936, you may be fascinated to learn—or be reminded—that as early as the late 1700s healers were making causal claims for specific methods that undoubtedly worked through common factors. Indeed, the history of psychotherapy in general and relationship therapy in particular is a history of growing awareness and appreciation (albeit only relatively recently for relationship therapies) of commonalities among change models.

Although much more has been written about common factors in the individual therapy literature, Chapter 3 focuses on four common factors that are unique to couple and family therapy: (1) conceptualizing difficulties in relational terms, (2) disrupting dysfunctional relational patterns disruption, (3) expanding the direct treatment system, and (4) expanding the therapeutic alliance. While few in number, these common factors are extremely important and rooted in the ways in which relationship therapy is itself distinctive.

Chapter 4 paints a "big picture" view of the major common factors (both "broad" and "narrow") that we believe drive change. Six categories of common factors are offered, along with an overview of the research evidence supporting them. This chapter sets the stage for Chapters 6–9, which present most of these categories in greater detail.

Chapter 5 focuses on our "moderate" view of common factors and how it differs from more radical versions that, among other things, suggest that models are irrelevant, impotent, or both. We articulate in greater depth our "both–and" position that values models but emphasizes that their major role is to activate common factors. Other common misconceptions (e.g., common factors are mostly about the therapeutic relationship) are also dispelled.

Specific Applications of Common Factors in Relational Therapy

Chapters 6–9 are the most practical sections of the book, offering many clinical examples. Chapter 6 looks at key "client" and "therapist" common factors and, specifically, how therapists can engage clients and match their level of motivation. The chapter applies Prochaska's (1999) transtheoretical stages of change and also Miller and Rollnick's (2002) motivational interviewing—two models traditionally used with individuals—as common factors lenses that can also inform relational therapy.

Chapter 7 hones in on the important therapeutic alliance—what it consists of and how it is formed, torn, and repaired—and the unique aspects of the alliance in couple and family therapy. Although most therapists think that they are skillful at building alliances, doing so successfully is a complex task requiring considerable skill, given both the unique alliance needs of specific clients and the pitfalls and intricacies of the multiple alliances in relational therapy.

Chapter 8 focuses on the unique relational common factor of interrupting dysfunctional relational patterns/cycles. What makes this chapter fascinating is that interventions from three seemingly disparate models (object relations, emotionally focused, and solution-focused) are shown to operate in similar ways as they interrupt the dysfunctional cycles of the same client couple. When one "stands meta" to (i.e., as though outside) these specific "different" interventions, it is clear that they utilize common principles of change.

Chapter 9 concludes this section by presenting a common factors meta-model of change for couple therapy. This "model of models" offers a guide to the change process irrespective of which relational model is being used. It integrates broad and narrow common factors into a coherent principle-based explanation of therapeutic change.

Conclusions, Implications, and Recommendations

Chapters 10–12 focus on conclusions, implications, and recommendations based on the common-factors-driven paradigm of change.

Although we are common factors proponents, we are also "evidence people" and thought we should also include a chapter (Chapter 10) on "The Case against Common Factors." Here we review the challenges to common factors and our responses to them. Chapter 11 discusses the implications of the common factors movement in relationship therapy for training and supervision. Our approach does not require educators to dramatically overhaul the content they teach, but it does have implications for both how models are viewed and how skills are taught in relation to one another. We also stress the need to learn multiple or flexible models because of the need to adapt to different types of clients. Finally, Chapter 12 offers specific recommendations to clinicians, supervisors, and researchers based on the ideas explored and explicated in this volume. We also use this opportunity to speak to the field of couple and family therapy.

Taken together, the chapters that follow add flesh to the bones of the contrast between the model-driven and the common-factors-driven paradigms of change set forth in Chapter 1. Hopefully, they will lead you, the reader, to think differently about, as well as weigh the implications of, our opening question, "What is responsible for therapeutic change?"

2

A Brief History
of Common Factors

Common factors play a crucial role in all psychotherapies, but their role often goes unnoticed or unacknowledged. Thus, it was not until 50 years after the beginnings of psychotherapy that the discourse about treatment began to include consideration of these factors. There are several possible reasons for this state of affairs, but we think that one emerges as most powerful and succinct. Model developers have largely been the leading writers and presenters in the field, and model developers and proponents have an intrinsic interest in highlighting the unique aspects of their approaches. In this regard, psychotherapies are not so different from other services and products in our society. Automobile advertisements, for example, don't speak to why it's good to have a car or why an automobile has a certain set of safety devices; rather, they underscore why, say, a Toyota is special and different from a Honda. It's left to *Consumer Reports* to tell us that Toyotas, Hondas, Lexuses, and other Japanese cars share much of the same technology.

In today's world of evidence-based behavioral practice, typically model developers simultaneously develop the treatments, disseminate the treatments, do the research on the treatments, evaluate the feasibility of grants to assess the impact of those treatments, and write the major reviews that evaluate those treatments. In such an environment, it is no great surprise that treatment differences are accentuated and brand names come to predominate. This trend is, if anything, even stronger in the world of couple and family therapies than in methods of individual therapy. Although there are many "named" individual therapies, these are typically subsumed within a broad approach to therapy. Thus, panic control therapy, the treatment developed by Barlow and Craske (Craske & Barlow, 2001) is often spoken of as cognitive-behavioral therapy for panic, though there also are several other unrelated cognitive-behavioral methods that deal with that problem or others. In contrast, in family therapy we today have five different but closely related models for the family treatment of adolescent substance use disorders, each separately named and evaluated and competing for adoption (Chamberlain, 2003; Henggeler, Schoenwald, Rowland, & Cunningham, 2002; Liddle & Rowe, 2002; Sexton & Alexander, 2005; Szapocznik et al., 2002).

Early School-Based Theories

There is an irony in common factors entering discourse about psychotherapy so late because before the beginnings of psychotherapy one well-known treatment that promised dramatic effects on functioning already had been notoriously exposed as stemming solely from the impact of common factors. Franz Anton Mesmer, the 18th-century German physician-performer, put forth a theory of "animal magnetism," in which he viewed health as being affected by the gravitational pull of the various planets. Mesmer traveled far and wide throughout Europe "curing" a wide range of illnesses through the practice of "mesmerism," which featured his passing magnets and his hands over people. In 1784, Louis XVI (who later was beheaded in the French Revolution) assembled a commission of scientists that included Benjamin Franklin to assess Mesmer's techniques. The commission concluded that, although some people felt better, these changes could in no way be related to Mesmer's specific techniques. The changes Mesmer described were unrelated to the techniques he employed or the theory he espoused. The changes that occurred could better be explained by the impact of the common factor of engendering hope and positive expectations in his patients than by the impact of his specific methods.

When Freud (1987) developed psychoanalysis as the first widely circulated psychotherapy, his focus was on articulating a specific theory of personality, psychopathology, and psychotherapy and elaborating specific methods of practice that fit with this theory and were effective in leading to change. Classic psychoanalysis first posited a specific treatment for a specific disorder, hysteria, and then expanded that technique to the treatment of other problems. As Jung (1916, 1935), Adler (1924/1957), and other theorists elaborated and debated what constituted the best methods of analysis, their focus too came to be on the theory of psychopathology and the various strategies in treatment. Jung emphasized a focus on the importance of the collective unconscious, Adler on feelings of inferiority, and each succeeding theory within the psychoanalytic school underscored a different emphasis. Although a reader today examining these approaches can readily see how these approaches invoke the common factors we describe in this book, these authors focused little if any attention in their writing or presentations on these factors.

During the era following World War II, this failure to focus on the commonalities that are present in all treatments was only further accentuated as therapies became increasingly diverse. Challengers began to emerge to the psychoanalytic paradigm, drawing from the quite distinct traditions of behaviorism (in such treatments as behavior therapy) and humanism (in such treatments as Gestalt and experiential therapies). The emerging books and presentations on how to do psychotherapy focused on identifying and debating what the key elements of human functioning were and how to change those factors, whether it be unconscious processes, behavior, cognitions, emotional life, or biology. Proponents of different approaches accentuated different levels of human experience, and even within these respective schools different specific approaches came to focus on differences in technique (e.g., as in the differences between rational-emotive [Ellis, 1962] and cognitive therapy [Beck & Weishaar, 1989] among the cognitive therapies). In this tradition of dueling therapies, little, if any, attention was directed toward what therapies shared.

First-Generation Family Therapies

Given the limited attention to common factors in therapies for individuals, it is remarkable that the first-generation couple and family therapies evidenced even less attention to these factors. Indeed, some of these early therapies promoted the extreme position of advocating deliberately *not* engaging in strategies that increase such common factors as positive expectancy and the therapeutic alliance described in this volume and specifically described tactics for *decreasing* these factors.

The Palo Alto variant of strategic therapy (Watzlawick, Weakland, & Fisch, 1974), a prominent set of methods in its time, called for exercising care to assure that the therapeutic alliance did not become too powerful. This approach utilized therapeutic directives coming from behind a one-way mirror to, in part, limit the connection between client and therapist, and called for an abrupt end to therapy when change occurred in order to avoid what was regarded as a dependency on the therapist as an agent of change. Another early therapy, Haley's problem-solving therapy (Haley, 1987), similarly emphasized reducing what we now know to be the common factor of creating positive expectancy in clients through focusing on paradoxical directives that promoted psychological resistance to the message of the therapist. These early systemic therapies had little faith in client resilience or an innate process of change, instead emphasizing homeostasis in systems and consequently methods through which a powerful strategic therapist could join with and trick the system into changing through such tactics as suggesting the family did not need to—or would not be able to—change.

Even when the message did not overtly undermine what we now regard as common factors, the first generation of approaches (as was true in individual therapies) focused on the unique value of the particular theory and the strategies of change within each school. Proponents of different theories argued the respective benefits of an emphasis on family structure, felt experience, differentiation of self, strategies of change, or object relations. Thus, Minuchin (1974) privileged structure and the use of enactments; Bowen (1972), coaching for interchanges within the family of origin; and Haley (1997), paradoxical directives. Books and presentations in the field focused on these theories and the methods of practice that flowed from them.

It is important to note that this dominant discourse about differences among theories and strategies for change among these family therapies obscured other commonalities that we can now see, with the passage of time, underlay these debates. Foremost, all these theories and approaches in family therapy centered on one shared vision, that of invoking social support and utilizing the family as a pathway to change. The strategies of intervention may have differed, but these approaches shared the common pathway of invoking change in family as a pathway toward other change.

Further, most of the early family therapies did agree about the importance of building alliance in some shape or form. For example,

Minuchin and Fishman (1981) devoted much of one volume to techniques for the practitioner's creating a therapeutic alliance with the family being treated; and Ackerman (1970), Bowen (1960), and Whitaker (Whitaker & Malone, 1953), and Boszormenyi-Nagy (Boszormenyi-Nagy & Spark, 1973) each allocated considerable attention to how to "join" with the family, that is, to create a therapeutic alliance. That these methods were presented as part of the core theory of practice in each school in languages that were unique to that school obscured the presence of underlying common factors applicable across all conjoint therapies.

Ultimately, the unique public demonstrations of the various approaches to family therapy in large workshops conducted around the world by the master therapists who were the founders of the schools of treatment offered an opportunity for those observing to begin to see common factors across the work of these therapists. When the actual work of these pioneers was observed, far more commonality was evident than might have been thought when first encountering descriptions of theory and strategy. Each of the charismatic generation of pioneers who developed focused theories and strategies clearly engaged in a much wider range of actual behavior in session than they spoke to in their writings, and all promoted closely connected human interaction in families as well as individual development. A research study during that time that examined the methods of these pioneers found significant overlapping in what they actually did in session (Pinsof, 1978).

Beginnings in the Understanding of Common Factors: Early Stirrings

Although the focus on differences in theory and strategy was the predominant paradigm in psychotherapy, there were early voices that began to talk about common factors as early as the 1930s. In the first prominent mention of such factors, Saul Rosenzweig (1936) published the earliest paper on common factors, suggesting that the effectiveness of psychotherapies stemmed more from their common elements than their specific methods. Specifically, Rosenzweig pointed to how each therapy centered on a relationship between client and therapist and each built on a theory of explanation. Rosenzweig also made the first reference to the "dodo bird verdict"—that therapies are roughly equal in outcome—described later in this chapter.

Jerome Frank

Despite Rosenzweig's (1936) work and that of a few other pioneers, it was only with the landmark work of Jerome D. Frank (1961) that a common factors viewpoint was brought fully to the attention of psychotherapists. In his bestselling volume *Persuasion and Healing*, Frank (coauthor with his daughter of the later editions of this work) looked to common threads that cross all efforts at healing, seeking to explain the impact of not only psychotherapy but also medicine and even traditional healers such as medicine men. He (Frank, 1973; Frank & Frank, 1991) identified four key aspects of such relationships: (1) an emotionally charged confiding relationship with a helping person, (2) a healing context, (3) a rationale that provides a plausible explanation for the client's problems and how to resolve them, and (4) a procedure that involves active participation of client and therapist and is believed by both to be a means of restoring health. It was these common elements (close confiding contact, a place that was agreed to be helpful, a shared rationale, and an agreed-upon frame for healing) that Frank suggested were the true foundations for change. Consistent with our own formulation, Frank suggested that therapist procedures matter, not because they are effective in and of themselves, but at least to a considerable degree because of the shared beliefs that they represent in suggesting the availability of paths to healing. Frank further argued that psychotherapy works principally because it helps to remoralize demoralized people, and that the generation of hope is ultimately the crucial ingredient in all psychotherapies, and for that matter, most other methods of healing.

Frank's work had considerable impact on the field of psychotherapy in its time. Although it certainly did not retard the movement to specific therapies (which continued—and still continue—to be created and augmented), it influenced the practice of many therapists and laid the foundation for today's integrative movement in psychotherapy.

Carl Rogers

Carl Rogers (Raskin & Rogers, 1989; Rogers, Kirschenbaum, & Henderson, 1989) brought another perspective to this conversation about shared elements. Rogers was the developer of a major school of treatment, person-centered therapy, in which he articulated a specific set of methods of treatment that he believed to be effective. In the language of today's evidence-based therapies, he created a manual-driven empirically supported treatment[1] based on a technology of empathic listening. Yet, Rogers's methods emphasized the common factor of the healing relationship and thereby also serve as a guide to all therapists about a transcendent set of principles of treatment. Rogers's notions of what constitutes a healing relationship by virtue of the personal qualities of the therapist now serve as the basis for most such concepts in the psychotherapy field as a whole.

Rogers suggested that there were three essential dimensions of the therapist that led to successful therapy: empathy, positive regard, and congruence. Empathy involves understanding the client's frame of reference and ways of experiencing the world. Rogers's concept of empathy focused on both cognitive and emotional understanding. He defined it as the therapist's sensitive ability and willingness to understand the client's thoughts, feelings, and struggles from the client's point of view—the ability to see completely through the client's eyes, to adopt his or her frame of reference (Rogers, 1957, 1961). He underscored the core importance of the therapist's capacity to take on the perspective of the client and express understanding and acceptance of his or her experience, an idea now almost universally accepted as a foundation of psychotherapy.

Rogers's second core aspect of the person of the therapist was positive regard (Farber & Lane, 2002). Rogers stated: "To the extent that the therapist finds himself (herself) experiencing a warm acceptance of each aspect of the client's experience as being part of that client, he is experiencing unconditional positive regard.... It means there are no conditions of acceptance.... It means prizing of the person.... It means caring for the client as a separate person" (Rogers, 1957, p. 101). Warmth is clearly part of this regard; at other points Rogers referred to "non-possessive warmth." Whether in a beginning trainee or veteran therapist, such an ability to convey respect and acceptance clearly represents a crucial aspect of successful psychotherapy.

---

[1]Ironically, Rogers's research-based therapies don't qualify for lists of empirically supported treatments (ESTs) today because the clients were not subjected to the kind of medical model-based assessment of their pathology that Rogers rejected as inconsistent with his approach. In all other ways, Rogers created a manual-driven treatment that was demonstrated to be effective in clinical trial research, the core criterion for determining which treatments qualify as ESTs. That a person-centered treatment cannot qualify for lists of ESTs because Rogers's research did not focus on a specific medical model-based diagnostic category is an indictment of the methods used in determining which therapies qualify as ESTs (see Chapter 11).

Rogers's third core aspect of the effective therapist he called "congruence" (Rogers, 1957). Congruence refers to the therapist's ability to freely and deeply be himself or herself. Rogers suggested that the therapist does not need to be able to remain congruent in all aspects of his or her own life, but pointed to the crucial importance of doing so in the therapeutic relationship. Rogers believed the therapist must be genuine and not deceive the client about his or her feelings. Although many models do not emphasize this quality in the therapist, few therapies are likely to be successful without the therapists remaining congruent.

Rogers's core set of therapist characteristics became prominent in the field of psychotherapy during the 1950s and 1960s as a byproduct of the popularity of his person-centered therapy (earlier called client-centered therapy). This level of attention to these factors initially declined after Rogers's death and the consequent reduction in training and practice in person-centered therapy that accompanied it. Nonetheless, although the specific model never regained widespread popularity, the basic importance of the ingredients Rogers emphasized has become part of the core of much psychotherapy (Norcross, 2002b). Furthermore, narrative, collaborative, and experiential models have emerged that contain Rogers's concepts at their center.

The Generic Model

Orlinsky and Howard (1987) added to the view of common factors in articulating what they called a "generic" view of psychotherapy. The generic model focused on core aspects of all psychotherapies, leaving room for each specific approach to treatment to be filled in within the context of the model. Orlinsky and Howard specified four generic frames within which psychotherapy could be considered.

The first of these, which they called "co-oriented activity," consists of the behavioral interactional aspects of social relations. This frame includes the therapist's behavior, the client's behavior, and the behavioral interaction between them. The Rogerian facilitative conditions (such as empathic listening) are examples of therapist behavior that fall into this category. Orlinsky and Howard suggested there also are a parallel set of generic client behaviors that matter in successful therapy, such as communicating about problems and expressing oneself.

The second frame, which they called "concurrent experience," includes the phenomenological perception of social events by the client, the therapist, and conjointly between client and therapist. Here, Orlinsky and Howard included client self-perceptions, client perceptions of the therapist, client perceptions of the therapeutic relationship, therapist perceptions of the client, therapist self-perceptions (for example, as competent or not), and therapist perceptions of the therapeutic relationship. Orlinsky and Howard viewed each of these factors in treatment as having enormous impact on the treatment that transcends the specific method.

The third generic frame, which they called "dramatic interpretation," includes the symbolic formulations of meaning and value that are made and communicated by participants in a relationship. This is the territory of meaning. What is the meaning of therapy for the client and the therapist? What does each of them view as the purpose of the treatment and his or her own sense of involvement?

The final frame suggested by Orlinsky and Howard, termed "regular association," encompasses the normative prescriptive patterns of relatedness that bind participants to the therapeutic relationship and includes such aspects as the frequency of meetings and the existence of a therapeutic contract about arrangements and confidentiality. These simple aspects of regular association—such as how long we meet, how often we meet, where we meet, and what the fee is—are rarely the center of attention in texts about treatments (indeed, we think that some of them, such as fees and fee collection, are almost never represented in treatment manuals within empirically supported treatments). Yet, they may have vast implications for treatment and represent a crucial core set of generic ingredients. For example, Orlinsky and Howard note that almost all psychotherapies are offered in units of 45 minutes to 1 hour and sessions are most often once per week, suggesting that there must be some underlying generic ingredient basic to psychotherapy at work here.

The major contribution of Orlinsky and Howard (1987) consists in calling attention to the many levels at which a therapy functions. Psychotherapy is both a shared experience between client and therapist—which has meaning in itself as a relationship—and a path to individual change for the client about the targets of that treatment. Orlinsky and Howard also called attention to such generic aspects of treatment as the therapeutic contract. Treatment contracts vary in expectations about length and the nature of what the client and therapist will do, but all treatments involve a contract (stated or unstated) that shapes the treatment, sometimes in significant ways.

Luborsky and the Dodo Bird Verdict

In one of the most commonly cited papers in psychotherapy Lestor Luborsky and his colleagues (Luborsky et al., 1975), analyzed the impact of various treatments on clients receiving those treatments. What emerged was what they termed the "dodo bird verdict" (a term borrowed from Rosenzweig and inspired by a passage in *Alice in Wonderland* where "everybody has won and all must have prizes"). They concluded that all treatments on average had the same level of effects, impacting positively in a substantial way on about three of every four clients. Basing their view on this analysis, Luborsky and colleagues concluded that the essence of treatments lies not in the specific methods highlighted in models but in the common factors that underlie all good treatments.

Luborsky's article has been the subject of much debate among researchers since its publication. The advocates of specific treatments that have been shown through research to be effective have questioned the "dodo bird verdict" of this research (Chambless, 2002). Yet, analysis (and reanalysis) of these data and the data subsequently accumulated as psychotherapy research has grown (to now thousands of studies) and continues to support this conclusion (Luborsky et al., 2002).

Karasu, Gurman, and Goldfried's Classifications of Change Agents

Several other insightful theorists have aimed to explicate the dimensions of change that underlie treatment models. Karasu (1986) regarded the specific interventions of particular psychotherapies as impacting the client by moving him or her to engage in one of three core processes: affective experiencing, cognitive mastery, or behavioral regulation. He suggested that, although the various approaches begin with different ideologies and strategies of change, each ultimately involves the client in one of these three core domains. For example, in psychoanalysis, the technique of free association invokes affective experiencing, interpretation invokes cognitive mastery, and reassurance promotes behavioral regulation. For Karasu, each therapy follows specific procedures to encourage clients to embrace similar goals and processes.

In a similar vein, Gurman (1978) explicated a set of mediating and ultimate goals of treatment that transcend the specific treatment approach undertaken. Mediating goals are short-term process goals within the treatment, whereas ultimate goals represent the ends sought in the therapy. Gurman laid out a classification scheme specifying which ultimate and mediating goals were invoked by each treatment approach, creating in the process a very comprehensive and cogent table. He found a great deal of overlap in the goals of the various approaches, especially when a common language was used to describe these goals.

In another highly influential contribution, Goldfried and Padaver (1982) differentiated among three levels of intervention in psychotherapy, namely, theories, strategies, and interventions. They argued that while therapists often act as if they are very different from one another because their theories differ, there remains a great deal of overlap among them at the level of strategies of change and interventions. For example, they suggest that although a cognitive therapist, an experiential therapist, and an analyst might differ considerably in how they envision the process of change, each may well help a client to engage in self-talk and to deepen his or her experience in the process of promoting therapeutic change.

Within the family field, Pinsof (1995) has created a matrix for describing intervention approaches, with the level of the system in focus in the problem and intervention (family, couple, individual, or larger system) specified along one axis and a meta-category describing the locus of the problem or intervention (e.g., behavioral, cognitive, emotionally focused, psychodynamic) along the other. And Breunlin, Schwartz, and Mac Kune-Karrer (1997) have suggested a number of meta-frameworks at work underlying the methods of family therapy, ranging from a focus on internal process to one on development and one on culture.

With the emergence of the integrative movement (discussed later in this chapter), there now are many such systems of classifying interventions into their core ingredients. Most of these systems appear to speak to the same core set of factors, described from slightly different points of view and with different language and divided in a slightly different way.

Results from Meta-Analyses of the Impact of Psychotherapy

Smith and Glass (1979) examined the impact of psychotherapy in the first major meta-analysis of psychotherapy outcomes. For readers not familiar with meta-analysis, it is a quantitative procedure that combines the results of many studies, typically by creating a common metric called an "effect size." Having a common metric is necessary since studies typically use different outcome measures and therefore comparing results is like comparing apples and oranges. The standardized difference between group means is the most common effect size. If a therapy approaches or achieves an effect size of 1.0 across many studies, this means that, on average, the mean of the treatment group is one standard deviation higher than the mean of the control group (Sprenkle, 2002). Smith and Glass (1979) found that psychotherapy did have a substantial impact. In research in which a group receiving psychotherapy and a control group not receiving it were compared, when the results of studies were summed, the difference between psychotherapy and control groups was statistically significant, having an effect size (0.84) that is statistically labeled a "large" effect. Translated into other terms, this means that about three of four treatment clients change more than control clients (to create some context for the meaning of these numbers, one should note that the relationship between smoking and cancer manifests a small effect size). The researchers also found no difference in effectiveness across treatments in their meta-analysis when mediating and moderating factors were controlled. A similar conclusion emerged in a subsequent meta-analysis of the impact of psychotherapy (Lambert & Ogles, 2004).

A quite similar conclusion emerged in a similar meta-analysis of couple and family therapy conducted by Shadish and colleagues (Shadish & Baldwin, 2002, 2003; Shadish et al., 1993; Shadish, Ragsdale, Glaser, & Montgomery, 1995; Sprenkle, 2002). Specifically, Shadish and his colleagues' work provided strong support for the conclusion that, although relational approaches have indisputable evidence for their effectiveness, there is almost no evidence that these approaches are differentially effective when compared to one another. Shadish et al. (1995) concluded: "Despite some superficial evidence apparently favoring some orientations over others, no orientation is yet demonstrably superior to any other. This finding parallels the psychotherapy literature generally" (p. 348). The researchers found it likely that the modest differences accounted for by approach may well be the result of confounds with other variables such as client characteristics. When they entered potential methodological confounds into a regression analysis, no effect was found for orientation at all. Similarly, Shadish and Baldwin (2002) concluded that "there is little evidence for differential efficacy among the various approaches to marriage and family interventions, particularly if mediating and moderating variables are controlled" (p. 365). Although some differences among treatments do show up in individual studies, these disappear in meta-analyses when confounds are controlled across large numbers of studies.

Lambert's Analysis

Beginning with the lens of looking to see how much various factors affect the outcome of psychotherapy, Michael Lambert articulated what is now the most widely disseminated way of classifying factors that affect treatment. Lambert divided the factors affecting treatment outcome into client factors, relationship factors, placebo factors, and treatment factors. Although the techniques that make up treatment factors are typically seen as the core set of ingredients in treatment, Lambert's reviews of empirical studies (Lambert, 1992; Lambert & Ogles, 2004) found such treatment factors to account for only a small percentage of the variance in studies of psychotherapy, a percentage dwarfed by client, relationship, and placebo factors. In his 1992 work, Lambert suggested that 40% of change occurring in treatment was attributable to extratherapeutic factors in the client's life (such as changing jobs, or life events that occur), 30% to relationship factors having to do with the alliance between the client and therapist, 15% to placebo factors or positive expectancy, and only 15% to the treatment intervention itself. Although the exact percentages of the variance accounted for by each of these factors has been much debated, Lambert's figures remain very influential. An important caveat is that his figures were estimates based on a literature review and were not formally mathematically derived. Thus, the most commonly accepted numbers, while admittedly inexact, do point to the preponderance of effects that stem from common factors while allowing for only a small impact from treatment factors.

In his analyses, Lambert (1992) also suggested that treatments do not vary much in their overall impact (in effect, reiterating the dodo bird verdict) and highlighted the strong evidence for the impact of the therapeutic alliance on outcomes. Lambert in his 1992 work also articulated yet another division of common factors into what he termed support factors, learning factors, and action factors. He suggested that the evidence points to a sequencing of these factors, with support setting the stage for learning, which in turn sets the stage for action.

The Great Psychotherapy Debate

Bruce Wampold (2001), in the widely circulated volume *The Great Psychotherapy Debate,* performed another meta-analysis of the impact of treatment and common factors on outcomes and arrived at an even more radical conclusion than Lambert, finding that treatment factors contributed almost nothing to outcomes. While Wampold's analyses have been questioned more than Lambert's, his bestselling book instantly transported his arguments for the limited impact of treatments and the crucial role of common factors from the relatively arcane world of psychotherapy researchers into the much wider discourse of practicing clinicians. Wampold made the crucial point that sometimes treatments claimed as effective are compared not to "bona fide" therapies widely practiced but rather to pseudotreatments that bear little resemblance to psychotherapy of any kind. For example, several studies have contrasted a therapy that was under review for empirical support with a version of humanistic therapy in which therapists simply limited their input to bland support and more repetition of client statements. When actual humanistic therapies, such as emotionally focused therapy, are studied, the rates of success are much different from those in these pseudotherapy versions of humanistic therapy. However, the major point of Wampold's book is that when treatments are compared with bona fide alternatives, his meta-analysis showed that data support the common factors paradigm. For example, effect sizes associated with the therapeutic alliance, therapist factors, and allegiance variables all trumped effect sizes associated with specific treatments.

The Heart and Soul of Change

Hubble and his associates (1999) followed these efforts with a major edited volume that included chapters examining each of the factors Lambert had designated and assessing the impact of common and treatment factors in different treatment contexts. The chapters in this volume suggested that the common factors, in Luborsky's words, take "all the prizes" in providing the essential impact of treatment. Like Wampold, Hubble et al. assumed what we call a radical view of common factors: that common factors wholly are the essence of psychotherapeutic treatment. Methods of intervention matter little, but what does matter is the generation of such aspects of treatment as a strong alliance and taking into account the vast importance of client factors (Duncan, Miller, & Sparks, 2004). They also placed great emphasis on the tracking of alliance factors and outcomes during the treatment to be sure it was being maximally effective.

As we have already noted, there is considerable debate about the numbers invoked by Wampold and Hubble and associates emerging out of meta-analyses for the relative contributions of treatment versus common factors that suggest the relatively trivial impact of specific treatments and treatment factors. Critics (Chambless, 2002; Wampold, Ollendick, & King, 2006) claimed that treatment factors account for more of the outcome in meta-analyses than common factors proponents would allow. These critics also argued that treatment factors tend to be underestimated in these meta-analyses (though we note here that even the most generous assessments fail to credit treatment factors for the most substantial part of the impact of therapy) because the treatments assessed in these meta-analyses are so diverse that the effects of treatment are lost. From the defenders' perspective, a better test of the impact of treatment factors would be to look at a more limited set of studies such as those comparing cognitive-behavioral treatments for treating anxiety disorders and other approaches.

As we discuss later (primarily in Chapters 5 and 11), we believe the correct balanced approach allows for acknowledging problems for which certain treatments work better than others as well as for those where treatment factors are unimportant—and "all must have prizes." Examples that emerge from the treatment research in which certain treatments do appear to have unique effectiveness for certain problems as compared to other treatments include sex therapy for sexual disorders (McCarthy, 2002), family psychoeducational treatments for schizophrenia (Anderson, Hogarty, & Reiss, 1980), and cognitive-behavioral treatments for panic disorder (Barlow, Pincus, Heinrichs, & Choate, 2003), obsessive–compulsive disorder (Franklin & Foa, 2007), and simple phobias (Barlow, Allen, & Basden, 2007).

However, the limited range of such findings must be juxtaposed against the wide array of problems and situations for which people seek therapy in which there are no similar results and where many treatments appear equally effective. For all of the more typical problems for which clients enter therapy, such as relationship problems, problems in living, and problems with self-esteem and depression, no one has yet demonstrated that treatment factors make much difference. Even if evidence-based ESTs can be created by showing that these treatments work, there is no reason to believe these treatments work any better than other treatments not yet subjected to research. What is missing from the literature is clear. No one has yet shown consistent treatment effects across studies comparing bona fide treatments aimed at these problems; and the number of research studies that have found that such bona fide treatments (when examined in relation to no treatment) don't work is very small, mostly concentrated in the treatment of a few difficult-to-treat problems.

The American Psychological Association Division of Psychotherapy Report

Recently, the Division of Psychotherapy of the American Psychological Association commissioned another volume examining which common factors have a sufficient empirical basis for their impact on outcomes to be regarded as established (Norcross, 2002b). This group found the therapeutic alliance, cohesion in group therapy, empathy, goal consensus, and collaboration to be well-established general elements in the therapy relationship. Looking at this list more specifically, the task force found overwhelming evidenciary support for the impact of the alliance between client and therapist on treatment outcome. In the group therapy context, they found that cohesion in the group (how members felt in relation to one another) had an analogous impact to that of the therapeutic alliance in individual therapy; that is, clients who feel connected to one another in group therapy generally have better outcomes. This task force also found that higher levels of therapist empathy led to better therapeutic relationships and outcomes, as did clients and therapists sharing the same goals for treatment. The task force also found that two ways of customizing the therapy to the individual client have been shown to have a favorable impact, namely, adapting the treatment to enable a better alliance with the client and adapting the treatment to the level of the functional impairment and the coping style of the client. In other words, considering carefully who the client is matters when framing a particular strategy of intervention.

The task force also identified a number of promising elements that had emerged from research but for which there were not as yet sufficient findings for these to be regarded as "well-established" relationship factors. These included positive regard and congruence (which we described earlier on our discussion of Carl Rogers); the feedback between client and therapist about progress; repairing alliance ruptures when the client comes to see the therapist in a negative light; therapist self-disclosure about his or her own life; the positive management of countertransference that arises in treatment; and offering relational interpretations about the relationship between client and therapist. Other factors identified as promising included adapting the therapy relationship to the individual client and his or her readiness to change (Prochaska, DiClemente, & Norcross, 1992), client expectations and preferences, client attachment style, client spirituality, and cultural diversity. In summary, the division task force made a strong case for the power of common factors in treatment and the potentially wide range of such factors.

The Integrative Movement in Psychotherapy and Family Therapy

In recent years a widespread movement has emerged within psychotherapy in general and more specifically within family therapy toward integration of treatments (Lebow, 2002). Any close observation of recent writing or clinical practice would suggest how completely the trend toward integration and eclecticism has transformed psychotherapy. Not only has a considerable literature emerged concerned with integration and eclecticism, but also numerous models have been developed and widely disseminated. Yet, oddly and perhaps emblematic of a paradigm shift, the move to integration and informed eclecticism has become so much part of the fabric of our work that it goes largely unrecognized.

There are many signs of this emerging paradigm. Methods often broach the boundaries of what earlier were distinct schools of psychotherapy (Goldfried & Norcross, 1995). The methods of "behavioral" therapists now often include strains of strategic therapy (Haas, Alexander, & Mas, 1988). "Cognitive" therapists pay far greater attention to affect than previously, and experiential therapists grapple with structure (Linehan et al., 1999). Work with "object relations" frequently involves the teaching of behavioral skills and pragmatic help in solving problems (Stricker & Gold, 2005). Articles and presentations refer again and again to a merging of concepts across diverse orientations.

Although professional identities continue to form within training programs grounded in schools of treatment and to be maintained despite the idiosyncratic pathways of professional development, actual methods of practice continue to broaden. While integrative and eclectic models in psychotherapy have existed for several decades, the extent of their acceptance is unprecedented. Surveys suggest that the great majority of practitioners identify themselves as integrative or eclectic in orientation (Norcross & Newman, 1992). Although new therapies, strategies, and techniques continue to be developed, the impact of these therapies often is greatest when concepts and interventions are integrated with more traditional methods. Little time passes between the development of an approach and its integration with other methods.

In today's clinical practice, even the broadest disjunction—that between "individual" and "couple" or "family" therapy—is regularly negotiated. Increasingly, interventions and precepts derived from individual therapy (e.g., cognitive-behavioral, psychodynamic, or self-psychology practices) are utilized in conjunction with systemic perspectives, and individual, couple, and family sessions are mixed freely in treatments. This is in marked contrast to early family therapy, whose practitioners criticized those who utilized concepts from individual therapy, asserting that the therapist was insufficiently systemic (Keith, Connell, & Whitaker, 1991; Minuchin, 1974), and to earlier individual-focused therapy, whose practitioners saw inclusion of family members as, at best, diluting the focus, and perhaps as harmful (through such mechanisms as undermining therapist–client transference).

A common language that transcends approach has begun to emerge as well as the beginnings of generic catalogs of interventions that transcend orientation. Several thoughtfully constructed integrative and systematic eclectic therapies also have been developed that have acquired considerable numbers of followers (Breunlin et al., 1997; Duncan, Sparks, & Miller, 2006; Liddle, Rodriguez, Dakof, Kanzki, & Marvel, 2005; Pinsof, 2005; Sexton & Alexander, 2003) and have helped popularize integrative and eclectic practice.

One major thread of integration consists in those approaches that highlight and emphasize common factors (Lebow, 2008). These methods focus primarily on the best implementation of common factors in psychotherapy, much as we do in this book. The emergence of the integrative/ informed eclectic paradigm probably was inevitable, but it was anticipated by few as arriving so quickly. Most therapists have switched from belaboring differences to instead focusing on integration in their practices.

Sprenkle and Blow's Moderate Common Factors Approach

Looking at the history of evidence described above and focusing on the role of common factors in the practice of marriage and family therapists, Sprenkle and Blow (2004a) articulated what they term a moderate common factors position. This position differed from the more extreme interpretations of common factors offered by Wampold (2001) or Hubble et al. (1999). From Sprenkle and Blow's (2004a) perspective, common factors are important, but one approach is not "just as good as another." They argue, instead, that it does matter what therapists do but that among effective psychotherapies there are only relatively small differences in treatment outcome. This view leaves room for the findings of clinical trial research as well as the meta-analyses that point to few differences in outcomes across treatments, as was described earlier. Sprenkle and Blow suggest that the contrast of common factors versus treatment factors need not be an either–or position. They allow for the likelihood of added specific benefit from treatment factors beyond that of common factors but want to be sure that common factors are accorded their rightful credit in treatment and in training.

Sprenkle and Blow (2004a) divide common factors into client factors, therapist effects, the therapeutic relationship, expectancy effects, and the nonspecific treatment variables described by Karasu (1986): behavioral regulation, emotional experiencing, and cognitive mastery. In the current volume we add a sixth miscellaneous category that includes allegiance effects and the organization or coherence of the model employed (see Chapter 4). In bringing the discourse about common factors into the domain of the practice of relational therapies, Sprenkle and Blow also added three common factors unique to relational therapies, namely, a relational conceptualization of problems, the expanded direct treatment system, and the expanded therapeutic alliance. These factors are described in detail in Chapter 3, where a fourth common factor is also discussed, namely, disrupting dysfunctional relational patterns.

The work of Sprenkle and Blow serves as much of the basis for this book. The publication of their paper in the *Journal of Marital and Family Therapy* (Sprenkle & Blow, 2004a, 2004b) led to an exchange of papers with Sexton, Ridley, and Kleiner (2004) in that journal debating the importance of common factors in couple and family therapy.

This chapter has traced the rich history of common factors.

While explicit mention of this term goes back to 1936 (Rosenzweig), the entire history of psychotherapy can be described as a dramatic conflict between the forces of specificity and commonality. Our commitment is to evidence. We believe that the evidence is more supportive of the common-factors-driven model of change, although we take a more moderate stance on this issue than some of our colleagues in the common factors camp. A detailed explanation of our "moderate" view will be offered in Chapter 5.

3

Common Factors Unique
to Couple and Family Therapy

The focus of this chapter is on common factors that are unique or distinctive to couple and family therapy. They are few in number, but we believe they are very important: (1) conceptualizing difficulties in relational terms, (2) disrupting dysfunctional relational patterns, (3) expanding the direct treatment system, and (4) expanding the therapeutic alliance.

That there are few distinctive common factors should not be too surprising since, at least numerically, the ways in which relational and individual psychotherapy are similar are much greater than the ways in which they are different. Both types of therapies, for example, rely heavily on the quality of the relationship between the therapist and the client(s). Both utilize change mechanisms that encourage clients to view their situations differently, to change dysfunctional behaviors, and to modify ways of expressing affect and to build stronger emotional connections.

It follows that almost all of what has been written about common factors in the individual psychotherapy literature applies to those who work with couples, families, and larger systems. Conversely, a great deal of what we say in the chapters that follow about common factors in relational therapy are just as applicable to work with individual clients (provided that the practitioner conceptualizes problems relationally; see below).

This overlap is fortunate since research designed to uncover common elements in the change process in individual psychotherapy has blossomed during the past 15 years (Davis & Piercy, 2007a). Virtually all of the now empirically well-grounded knowledge from individual psychotherapy research about common factors (for example, the importance of therapist competence, independent of the model employed) undoubtedly applies to all relational therapy approaches. Research on specific common factors in couple and family therapy remains in its infancy, leading Davis and Piercy (2007a) to conclude that we have much less direct empirical evidence about common factors that are unique to psychotherapy with larger systems than with individuals. However, as we shall see shortly, there is strong indirect evidence for the first two of the four unique common factors and fairly strong direct evidence for the third.

So, just as there are some important ways in which couple and family therapies are distinctive from individual psychotherapies, there are common factors that are unique to relational therapies that we believe are crucial.

Conceptualizing Difficulties in Relational Terms

One distinctive common element in all larger system therapies is conceptualizing human difficulties in relational terms. This element stands in sharp contrast to the DSM view that mental disorders are conditions that occur "within a person."

If Jamaal (age 35 years) is depressed, relationship therapists would not deny "within-person" elements like reduced serotonin (biology) or cognitive distortions (psychology) since they value a biopsychosocial (Engle, 1977) approach. However, Kayla, his relationship therapist, would be much more likely to view Jamaal's malady within the context of his social network, paying particular attention to the complex web of reciprocal influences contributing to the complaint. This view would lead Kayla to keep the whole system (or systems) in view when interacting with any part of the system (Wampler, 1997). So, for example, Kayla might pay attention to Jamaal's problematic relationship with his employer while at the same time paying attention to patterns or expectations about work that derived from his family of origin, where occupational success was highly valued. Kayla, herself an African American, would certainly take into account the race of her client (also African American) and what it was like for him to work in a predominantly white company. Jamaal's cognitive distortions (for example, his perfectionism) would also be conceptualized as both influenced by and influencing his social interactions and cultural environment. Moreover, Kayla would attempt to relate in a positive way to all elements of the system(s) irrespective of who happens to be in the therapy room (Wampler, 1997). So, for example, if Jamaal's wife, Samantha, happened to refuse treatment (which she did not), Kayla would still consider her to be very much "present" in the treatment, as she would also with Jamaal's boss and colleagues at work since they were part of the relationship therapy conceptualization of Jamaal's depression (Sprenkle, Blow, & Dickey, 1999). Pinsof (1995) calls the cast of characters who are important to treatment and yet not physically present the "indirect" treatment system.

Another way of stating this unique common factor is that relational therapies pay special attention to the interactional cycles among the various subsystems that constitute the larger system in which the problem is embedded.

The research of Davis and Piercy (2007a, 2007b) offers empirical support for this common factor. They found that the developers of three different relationship therapy models (emotionally focused therapy, cognitive-behavioral couple therapy, and internal family systems therapy), their students, and the clients of both groups tended to view the success of treatment in couple therapy similarly. Therapy worked, in part, because the therapists got the clients to see the problems in terms of dysfunctional interactional cycles.

Davis and Piercy (2007a, 2007b) were more specific in that they found that proponents of each of the models emphasized that these patterns were learned in the family of origin of clients and that each model conceptualized the cognitive, affective, and behavioral components that perpetuated the current interactional cycle. These commonalities were somewhat surprising since some of these models (e.g., cognitive-behavioral couple therapy and emotionally focused therapy) are not typically viewed as emphasizing the family of origin. Furthermore, several of the models are typically seen as specializing in one domain (e.g., emotionally focused therapy on emotion); yet the data showed that each model gave attention to the cognitive, affective, and behavioral dimensions of dysfunctional cycles—even though it might specialize in one domain.

Earlier we noted that there was strong indirect evidence for this common factor. Quantitative researchers have rarely directly tested "relationship conceptualization" versus "no relationship conceptualization" in randomized clinical trials (which is not the same thing as comparing relationships as the unit of treatment versus individuals as the unit of treatment—as will be elaborated later). Nonetheless, it is universally true that all of the strongly empirically validated relationship therapy approaches employ a relationship conceptualization of the problems they are addressing. Since interventions based on this way of looking at difficulties are associated with such strong results (Pinsof & Wynne, 1995; Shadish & Baldwin, 2002; Sprenkle, 2002), we believe the indirect evidence for relationship conceptualization is powerful. For example, based on 20 meta-analyses in the couple and family therapy research literature, Shadish and Baldwin (2002) indicate that the average effect size for couple therapy is 0.84 and the average for family therapy is 0.58. That puts couple therapy on a par with the effect size for coronary bypass surgery, which is 0.80 (Shadish & Baldwin, 2002, p. 348); both are considered strong effect sizes. The effect size for family therapy is considered a moderate effect size, perhaps lower than couple therapy because the former has tended to be applied to more difficult multiproblem cases. By way of comparison, the effect size for AZT treatment of AIDS, also considered "moderate," is 0.47 (Shadish & Baldwin, 2002, p. 348).

Disrupting Dysfunctional Relational Patterns

Davis and Piercy (2007a) also concluded that therapists help their clients to interrupt or disrupt dysfunctional relational cycles. We believe that historically relationship therapists have almost always viewed their work as breaking up the dysfunctional or pathological interactional cycles that keep couples, families, and larger systems "stuck." Structural family therapists, for example, view their interventions as disrupting dysfunctional patterns of family organization (Minuchin, 1974); strategic therapists (Haley, 1987), as breaking up behavior sequences; Bowen (1978) therapists, as blocking triangulation or other intergenerationally transmitted patterns; Palo Alto systems therapists (Fisch, Weakland, & Segal, 1983), as blocking dysfunctional attempted solutions; emotionally focused therapists (Johnson, 1996), as interrupting persistent pathological emotional patterns; and so forth. So, it is safe to say that disrupting dysfunctional relationship patterns is the curative common factor flipside of relational conceptualization. While practitioners of individual therapy might say that they disrupt patterns too, we are talking here about the specific relational patterns that are the essence of the relational conceptualization of problems in couple and family therapy.

Davis and Piercy (2007a, 2007b) also found that, as with relational conceptualization, all the therapists in their study, regardless of model preference, used cognitive, behavioral, and affective interventions to interrupt cycles—even though emotionally focused therapists tended to specialize in emotional interventions and cognitive-behavioral couple therapists emphasized cognitive and behavioral procedures. For them, a common intervention factor in the therapies they studied was a tripartite range of mechanisms to interrupt dysfunctional patterns.

It remains to be seen whether Davis and Piercy's (2007a, 2007b) more specific findings about interactions cycles—first, that they are always rooted in the family of origin of the clients, and second, that they always contain affective, cognitive, and behavioral conceptual and intervention dimensions—will be true of all relational therapies. We suspect, however, that at least the second of these more specific findings is a common factor in all couple and family therapies.

As with relationship conceptualization, the indirect evidence for disrupting dysfunctional relational patterns is strong. All of the best empirically validated approaches to relational therapy utilize interventions that are focused on pattern disruption (Sprenkle, 2002).

Expanding the Direct Treatment System

Most relationship therapists push to involve more than the identified patient (or in some cases the willing participant) in therapy. Pinsof (1995) distinguishes between persons physically present in treatment ("direct patient systems") and those involved via the aforementioned "indirect systems." It is important to note that some important larger system issues such as gender, race, and culture usually impact both the indirect and direct treatment systems. While relational therapies almost always pay attention to indirect systems in case conceptualization, most practitioners believe that the power at the heart of couple and family therapy resides in the live systems "directly" present in the consulting room. So, although Jamaal was the person presenting with depression, Kayla would likely include Jamaal's spouse, Samantha, in at least some of the sessions to assess the extent to which Jamaal's depression was embedded in the spousal subsystem or perhaps masking a primary relational issue. Kayla might also include the couple's two children, Elijah, 13, and Belinda, 15, to gain a sense of how the adult issues were impacting the children, to check out whether parenting or child behavioral issues were impacting the problem, and to assess whether improving broader system dynamics might diminish pain in the family.

Pinsof (1995) suggests that there are five main reasons for adopting an "interpersonal premise," or bias, in favor of expanding the direct treatment system.

1. "Therapists will generally learn more about patient systems if they meet as many of the key patients as possible" (Pinsof, 1995, p. 98). The therapist gets a clear impression of the interpersonal dimensions of the patient system (Sprenkle et al., 1999).
2. "The therapist usually will establish a stronger therapeutic alliance with the patient system if that alliance is based on face-to-face contact" (Pinsof, 1995, p. 98).
3. "Doing as much of the work as possible in front of the key patients maximizes the likelihood of creating a wider, more stable, and more empathic collective observing ego" (Pinsof, 1995, p. 98). By this, Pinsof means that more people understand what is happening and why it is happening; and if one person loses perspective, another participant may be able to help him or her regain it (Sprenkle et al., 1999).
4. "The transforming impact of major breakthroughs is usually greater when they occur in the presence of key patients" (Pinsof, 1995, p. 99).
5. "The therapist will have a more accurate understanding of the problem maintenance structure if key patients are directly involved in ongoing treatment" (Pinsof, 1995, p. 99). Pinsof defines "problem maintenance structure" as all of the "constraints" (be they organizational, biological, emotional, cognitive, family of origin, object relations, or issues of the "self") that prevent family members from resolving their issues (Sprenkle et al., 1999).

While Pinsof qualifies these propositions—depending on variables like the type of family in therapy, the stage of treatment, and the types of issues being discussed—and he calls for a flexible approach that may emphasize the presence of different subsystems (and individuals alone) at certain times in treatment, nevertheless he clearly emphasizes including the "key players" at least some of the time. We agree, and we see the "interpersonal premise" as a key common factor that is unique to couple and family therapy.

Probably most relationship therapy practitioners, regardless of orientation, can readily recount times when the "common factor" of including more people in the direct client system was central to achieving positive results (Sprenkle et al., 1999). While there is little direct research evidence for these specific interpersonal premises, there is strong evidence that for a number of problems conjoint approaches are generally more successful than individual therapy for the same issue. For example, the evidence is strong for general marital dysfunction (Johnson, 2002), adolescent treatment of conduct disorders (Henggeler & Sheidow, 2002), adolescent treatment of substance abuse (Rowe & Liddle, 2002); couple versus individual treatment of alcoholism and adult drug abuse with behavioral couple therapy (O'Farrell & Fals-Stewart, 2002), and family management of severe mental illness (McFarlane, Dixon, & Lucksted, 2002).

Looking at these three common factors together (relationship conceptualization, pattern disruption, and the expanded direct treatment system), there is some tension within the ranks of relational therapists regarding whether all models capitalize fully on these common factors. For example, at the 1997 annual meeting of the American Association for Marriage and Family Therapy, Augustus Napier (1997) questioned whether some of the social constructionist models like narrative therapy or collaborative language systems were truly relational therapies since they place so much emphasis on changing how individuals view their situation. Salvador Minuchin (1998), in his provocative paper "Where Is the Family in Narrative Family Therapy?," also asserted that these models do not sufficiently emphasize the transactions among family members:

> Instead of observing the way in which family members affect each other in their transactions, creating patterns that enhance and constrain the views of self and others, these narrativists tend to privilege the discourse of individual members. Other family members are made the audience. The systemic idea that family members co-construct meaning, and that one can observe them in the process of constructing individual and family stories, is lost. The family, that natural interpersonal context in which people develop their views of themselves in the world, disappears from practice. (p. 399)

In their response to Minuchin, narrative therapists Eugene Combs and Jill Friedman (1998) emphasize that, *by not attending* to typical family transactions, the therapist actually interrupts these dysfunctional cycles:

In our early experience of doing family therapy, when we did encourage family members to talk and interact directly with each other, people often listened from a defensive position, planning their responses to each other's accusations rather than fully attending to the person speaking. In their interactions, they reenacted the problems that come to therapy. We have come to believe that these enactments tended to reinforce and strengthen the problems. We have found that inviting people to assume a witnessing position to each other's new stories frees them to hear instead of to defend. Hearing things differently and giving voice to these differences contributes to transformation. (p. 407)

In spite of their differences, once again both sides in this debate seem united in the belief that the role of the therapist is to break up dysfunctional cycles. These debates will probably continue since they are rooted in controversies regarding how family problems begin, are maintained, and are best addressed.

There is also little research on the extent to which direct conjoint participation adds to relationship conceptualization. Most comparisons are between conjoint and individual treatment modalities rather than between relationship conceptualization and individual conceptualization. We are aware of only two studies, both by Jose Szapocznik and colleagues (Szapocznik, Kurtines, Foote, Perez-Vidal, & Hervis, 1983, 1986) that contrasted "individual" (yet with a relational conceptualization) family therapy with a conjoined approach (that is, similar assumptions but a different unit of treatment). These investigators compared a conjoint version of structural family therapy with a single-person model—typically the drug-abusing adolescent. Both approaches significantly (but not differentially) reduced adolescent drug use and improved family functioning in the Hispanic families studied, but the single-person version produced better long-term results. These studies, however, employed small sample sizes, were ethnically homogeneous, and used a single theoretical orientation; so, it would be premature to generalize from them (Sprenkle et al., 1999).

On the other hand, given the aforementioned large body of research contrasting individual versus conjoint treatment approaches, which is favorable for conjoint approaches in multiple areas, we can say there is significant direct evidence for this common factor. However, it is not clear how many of these "individual" treatments utilized a systemic conceptualization. Probably most relational therapy practitioners, for example, have enjoyed some success treating couples with an absent partner; so, it is likely that the issue is quite complex and not all of pertinent variables have been teased out and researched (Sprenkle et al., 1999).

Expanding the Therapeutic Alliance

The alliance between the client and the therapist will be the specific focus of Chapter 7. Suffice it to say here that the alliance is one of the most potent common factors and one for which there is strong empirical support. It is also a somewhat complex topic since the alliance is believed not only to include the emotional "bond" or connection between the therapist and client(s) but also to encompass the extent to which clients and therapists are on the same page regarding the "goals" of therapy as well as the methods or activities employed in the therapy (the "tasks"). Since the alliance will be treated in more detail later, we will focus here only on the "bonds" component—the extent to which the client (especially) and therapist feel understood and emotionally connected.

While the alliance is important in all therapies, when more than one person is involved in the direct client system there is an expanded therapeutic alliance (or set of alliances) that is a common factor unique to couple and family therapy. When Jamaal, Semantha, Elijah, and Belinda participate in treatment, each of the four individuals will have an alliance with the therapist. Jamaal, for example, may have a strong personal "bond" with the therapist, but Elijah may not. In addition, however, each subsystem (parents, the couple, and the siblings) will also have a separate subsystem alliance that may be distinctive from the individual alliances (Pinsof, 1995). For example, Jamaal may feel positively about his personal alliance with Kayla but not believe that she is well aligned with him and Semantha as a couple. Or Elijah might not feel personally understood by Kayla but might feel that she is supportive of his and Belinda's rights, as siblings, to more privileges vis-à-vis their parents as the teenagers take on more responsibility. That is, Elijah may feel good about Kayla's understanding of the needs of the sibling subsystem. Furthermore, the entire family may have an alliance with the therapist that is more than the individual and subsystem alliances combined (Pinsof, 1995). Perhaps, for example, family members as a unit believe that Kayla has a pretty good grasp of their broad family dynamics and that the sessions do facilitate their communicating better and everyone's taking some responsibility for the family's issues. This may be true despite family members' concerns about Kayla's alliance with some of them as individuals or as subsystems.

It seems likely that synergies operate here. If Jamaal, Samantha, Elijah, and Belinda all experienced their therapist, Kayla, as warm, empathic, and understanding—and they feel this bonding not only as individuals but also in their roles as part of subsystems as well as the whole family—then the therapy should get a powerful boost. This same kind of positive synergy is also possible for the goals dimension and the tasks dimension of the alliance.

Of course the expanded therapeutic alliance is a two-edged sword. If there is a "split" alliance—say, the parents bond well with the therapist but the teenagers bond poorly—then the advantage of broadening the direct system may turn into a liability. Since not all alliances are equally important, the extent of the damage would depend upon the centrality of the teenagers to the problem for which the family sought treatment and the power of the teenagers to sabotage therapy.

While there is plenty of research evidence on the importance of the alliance in relationship therapy (see Chapter 7), there is not much data yet regarding the multiple alliances described above. For this reason, we are more tentative about this last of the four unique common factors in couple and family therapy. There is some evidence that split alliances are deleterious and that having a balanced alliance with various family members may be more important than the strength of the alliances per se (Hollander-Goldfein, 1989; Pinsof, 1995; Sprenkle & Blow, 2004a). In any event, research in this area is still in its infancy.

Before concluding this section, we wish to acknowledge that relationship therapists, by virtue of their systemic conceptualization, may also have a unique "alliance" with the indirect treatment system in some cases. If a couple and family therapist, for example, treats a school-phobic child and his parents, and conceptualizes the school as part of the indirect treatment system (school representatives never actually attend sessions), this therapist may establish an alliance with the school either indirectly through the clients or through telephone calls or correspondence. Feeling valued by the therapist, even indirectly, might motivate school personnel. Presumably a nonsystemic therapist who conceptualized the child's problem intrapsychically would not have such an alliance and its potential salutary effect.

In this chapter we have described four common factors that are unique to couple and family therapy. The reader will note that they are part and parcel of what distinguishes relational therapies from individual therapies. We believe that there is sufficient research evidence (indirect but powerful for the first two and direct for the third) to say that at least the first three common factors are key to the efficaciousness of couple and family therapy. That the therapeutic alliance is also a powerful component of the success of relational therapy is also indisputable. Future research will determine the evidence for the impact of the multiple alliances that we described.

4

The Big-Picture View
of Common Factors

The earth looks a lot different from 60,000 feet than from 5,000 feet. In this chapter we will give a big-picture view of common factors, describing the major categories. We will hone in on the clinical implications in the chapters that follow, especially Chapters 6–9, which are rich with clinical illustrations of the concepts presented here.

The reader will recall that in Chapter 1 we made a distinction between the broad view and the narrow conceptualization of common factors. The former view includes all dimensions of the treatment setting that contribute to treatment outcome, including, for example, client and therapist variables, whereas the narrow view focuses on the commonalities among the interventions used by the proponents of therapy models. The narrow definition is only one part of the larger picture. The various dimensions of the broad definition of common factors, then, will be our focus here.

In the first chapter we also discussed that what you "see" regarding the process of change depends upon your particular paradigm, or the set of lenses through which you view psychotherapy. For most of our careers, the three of us authors saw psychotherapy through the model-driven change paradigm, and it did not even occur to us that the unique and/or particular dimensions of models might not be the primary engines that drive change. As we describe the major categories of common factors here, it is now somewhat hard to believe that we did not give more attention to these common factors since, "post-paradigm shift," they now seem relatively obvious.

Interestingly, Saul Rosenzweig, the founding father of common factors, said over 70 years ago that *"unrecognized factors* in a therapeutic situation may be much more important than those to which we pay attention" (1936, p. 412). People focused unduly on the specifics of models, he was arguing, not the unrecognized common factors. This same way of viewing change has marked most of the history of couple and family therapies until recently.

Of course, the common factors "in our sight" now are hardly the final picture, and so, as we begin our portrait of the common factors below, we readily acknowledge that future research will likely discover other "unrecognized factors" that are not yet apparent.

Based on current knowledge, we believe there are six major categories of common factors.

Client Characteristics as Common Factors

That the characteristics of the client should contribute mightily to the outcome of psychotherapy is especially self-evident post-paradigm shift. How could we have previously paid such little attention to them? Perhaps this oversight is due to what Tallman and Bohart (1999) refer to as psychotherapy's "professional centrism," or the self-referential tendency of highly trained professionals to think in terms of what *our* models, *our* techniques, and *our* skills accomplish. Recall from Chapter 1 that the client's role in the process of change is one of the major dimensions that distinguishes the model-driven from the common-factors-driven paradigm. Although there is variability since the two paradigms are not polar opposites, and some model-driven proponents work collaboratively, overall they are more likely to view the therapist as performing a treatment "on" clients and/or guiding them from the vantage point of an "expert."

Perhaps one of the major contributions of the common factors movement is highlighting the truth that the client, rather than the model or the therapist, is probably the major "hero" in change (Duncan & Miller, 2000). As Beutler, Bongar, and Shurkin (1998) put it, "If we look at factors contributing to the success of treatments, it is not the clinician or treatment procedure that is key, but the motivation, awareness, expectations, and preparation of the patient or client" (p. 8). To their list of desirable client characteristics or qualities we would certainly add the attribute of "hard work."

Tallman and Bohart (1999) offer a useful metaphor to drive home this point. Clients go to a health club to achieve a goal like cardiovascular fitness. The health club offers a variety of methods to facilitate its clients achieving these goals—such as treadmills, stationary bicycles, elliptical trainers, and stair-stepper machines. Now, what matters most? Is it the choice of machine that is crucial or, rather, the willingness of the client to get out of bed, go down to the club, and work hard and faithfully? Clearly the latter is more essential. While the machines certainly help to achieve the goal of cardiovascular fitness, the clients' engagement, motivation, and tenacity all trump the choice of machine (or, by analogy, therapy models).

Tallman and Bohart (1999) believe the reason that a number of psychotherapy models work approximately equally well is because clients have a unique ability to take whatever is offered by the therapist and use it for their own individual purposes. The research by Helmeke and Sprenkle (2000) on pivotal moments in couple therapy supports this conclusion. These investigators asked clients and therapists after each session whether anything happened that they considered "pivotal" and, if so, what it was. Helmeke and Sprenkle (2000) found out that clients often reconstructed events in the sessions for their own purposes, and *typically* what they thought was pivotal was different than what the therapist thought was pivotal in the same session. All three of us authors have had the humbling experience of asking clients for feedback about their evaluation of sessions, or the course of therapy (parts of us probably hoping for adulation for our "great work"), only to be deflated. The clients seized on something we considered a minor theme, or even misinterpreted us and noted something we would never say was pivotal, or they referred to an event outside of therapy, like getting a new job, that made a big difference for them.

Michael Lambert (1992) was among the first scholars to draw attention to the important role of the client in accounting for the outcome variance in psychotherapy. He, however, used a more narrow definition of "common factors" and did not apply this label to the client's contribution, even though he was quite specific that this contribution was independent of the therapy model employed. Furthermore, it was clear that he believed client factors (including motivation, commitment to change, inner strength, and religious faith), along with what he called extratherapeutic factors (such as social support, community involvement, stressful events, or serendipitous occurrences) accounted for the largest portion of the variance in outcome (40% by his estimate—or "guesstimate," since this percentage was not mathematically derived). Hubble et al. (1999) modified Lambert's model and called the same variables common factors. These authors took pains to stress that, when combined with the therapeutic relationship, a substantial portion of outcome variance—perhaps as much as 70%—was not directly under the therapist's control. Whatever the exact percentage may be, several other scholars (Beutler et al., 1998; Sprenkle & Blow, 2004a; Tallman & Bohart, 1999) share the conclusion voiced by Miller, Duncan, and Hubble (1997) that "the research literature makes it clear that the client is actually the single, most potent contributor to outcome in psychotherapy" (pp. 25–26).

Given this importance, it is unfortunate that most of the research in relational therapy related to clients focuses on the static characteristics of individuals such as age, gender, race, and sexual orientation. There is virtually no research on client characteristics much more likely to be strongly related to outcome—such as motivation for, and engagement in, treatment; perseverance and cooperation in completing homework assignments; and so forth (Sprenkle & Blow, 2004a) One study by Holtzworth-Munroe, Jacobson, Deklyen, and Whisman (1989) offers some evidence that these variables are significant contributors. The research of Prochaska (1999) on client motivation for change is well known in the literature on therapy for individuals, but we know of no empirical test in the relationship literature. We do, however, apply (theoretically) this model to couple and family therapy in Chapter 6.

Finally, there has been an unfortunate tendency within psychotherapy research to focus on client diagnosis (and clients are often considered homogeneous within DSM categories) "while ignoring the idiosyncratic aspects of the client that are even more salient in predicting change and guiding treatment decisions" (Clarkin & Levy, 2004, p. 195). Too often in clinical trials research clients' individual differences are considered a source of "error" rather than an opportunity for discovery. There are, however, a few examples where couple and family therapy model developers have provided evidence regarding the types of clients for whom their models we may be most appropriate or effective. Johnson and Talitman (1997) stated that emotionally focused therapy worked best for couples who thought the "tasks" of therapy that emphasize creating emotional connection are relevant and on target; and Jacobson and Christensen (1996) reported that traditional behavioral marital therapy is most successful for couples with high partner commitment, low "traditionality," and mutually agreed-upon goals for the marriage. We hope there will be much more research on significant client variables as common factors in the future. While we accept the consensus of common factors scholars that client variables are probably the most potent of the common factors categories, the empirical case is underdeveloped.

Therapist Characteristics as Common Factors

Recall that in Chapter 1 we said that the therapist's role in the process of change was also one of the major factors that made the two paradigms distinct. Although intuitively also appealing (common sense suggests that some therapists consistently get better results than others), the empirical evidence for therapist characteristics as significant common factors is much stronger. Unfortunately, however, although we can say unequivocally that therapist competence independent of models makes a major contribution to therapy outcome, we know too little about *why*. What specific aspects of competence make a difference?

First, let's take a look at the evidence for the overall conclusion. Arguably, the best, most comprehensive, and most impartial psychotherapy study ever completed was the National Institute of Mental Health (NIMH) Collaborative Depression Study (Elkin et al., 1989). Unlike most psychotherapy studies, which typically are completed by the founders of particular models or their colleagues or students, this study had no particular ax to grind. The therapists in this large multisite trial were trained to reach high standards of adherence to a manualized treatment for depression (cognitive-behavioral or interpersonal psychotherapy) as well as an antidepressant drug treatment condition and an attention placebo clinical management condition. The therapists in each group were equally highly experienced and had an allegiance to the model they utilized. In spite of strong efforts to control therapist factors, the results demonstrated that there were major differences in therapist effectiveness even though there were only minor differences in outcomes among the treatment models (Blow, Sprenkle, & Davis, 2007).

In a secondary analysis, Blatt, Sanislow, Zuroff, and Pilkonis (1996) divided the therapists into less effective, moderately effective, and more effective groups based on a composite outcome score for clients in each condition. The investigators found that "significant differences exist in the therapeutic efficacy among therapists, even with the experienced and well-trained therapists in the [NIMH] study" (p. 1281). These differences also turned out to be independent of the treatment model, the setting, and even the experience level of the clinician. Perhaps most surprisingly, Blatt et al. (1996) reported that the most favorable results were achieved by a female psychiatrist who saw clients only in the antidepressant drug clinical management and placebo (half her cases) clinical management condition, and not in either the cognitive-behavioral therapy or interpersonal therapy conditions. They remarked:

> It is noteworthy that this therapist's high level of therapeutic effectiveness was accomplished while seeing patients for a relatively brief time each week (approximately 25 minutes) as part of ... a procedure designed as a minimal therapeutic condition to provide only therapeutic support and encouragement. (p. 1281)

These conclusions led Blow et al. (2007) to conclude that "the history of the NIMH Depression study may prove to say more about 'empirically validated therapists' than about empirically validated therapies!" (p. 302).

Other important evidence comes from the book *The Great Psychotherapy Debate* (Wampold, 2001), based on a major meta-analysis of psychotherapy studies, all of which included a comparison among bona fide treatments. Wampold devoted an entire chapter to how therapist factors contribute to outcome variance in psychotherapy. Wampold presents convincing statistical evidence that differences among therapists contribute more (an effect size of 0.60) than the treatments they practice (which is at most 0.20 but probably closer to zero). Furthermore, when therapist variability is ignored, this significantly inflates Type I errors and makes treatments look more different than they actually are. The research of Wampold (2001) and Blatt et al. (1996) confirms earlier work by Luborsky et al. (1986), who examined data from four major psychotherapy projects and also concluded that therapist effects exceeded treatment effects. While not all studies have shown significant therapist variability, clearly the preponderance of the evidence supports the major conclusion of the studies just reviewed. Furthermore, since it is highly likely that there is greater therapist variability in the general population of practitioners as compared to therapists in research studies, this conclusion is likely to be even more valid in the "real world."

However, as noted previously, although the evidence for variability is powerful, we know surprisingly little about why the variability exists—apart from the fact that some therapists achieve strong relationships (therapeutic alliances with clients) and others do not. We will be treating the therapeutic alliance as a separate category below and also in great detail in Chapter 7.

In the research just reviewed, high therapist competence was operationalized as simply getting good results. We probably know relatively little about the specifics of competence or expertise since there has been relatively little research on this issue as compared to research on treatments. Recall that in Chapter 1 we noted that model-driven change places very little emphasis on therapist factors since *who* delivers the treatment is regarded as relatively unimportant. Models are studied like "drug research without the drugs." Beutler, Malik, and Alimohamed (2004) argue that over the past two decades the emphasis on randomized clinical trials focused on comparing models has actually resulted in *less* attention to therapist variables. These authors state:

> In efficacy research, the focus is on maximizing the power of treatments. Thus, efforts are made to control the influences of therapist factors by constructing treatment manuals that can be applied in the same way to all patients within a particular diagnostic group, regardless of any particular clinician. This research gives scant attention to any curative role that might be attributed to therapist factors that are independent of the treatment model and procedures. (p. 227)

Hence, therapist effects are treated as sources of error rather than sources of the variance, so that change can be attributed to the treatment model. However, as previously noted, there is compelling evidence that therapist variability exists even in highly controlled investigations (Blow et al., 2007). As Beutler et al. (2004) put it, "Unfortunately, standardizing the treatment has not eliminated the influence of the individual therapist on outcomes" (p. 245).

Aside from the therapist's contribution to the therapeutic alliance (to be covered later), here is a brief summary of what we know about the specifics of therapist variables, with a special emphasis on relational therapy. At the outset, we note that most of the variables studied do not contribute greatly to outcome (in terms of meta-analysis, many of these variables have small effect sizes). There is much that we do not know. First, as was true with client variables, "static" therapist variables such as the therapist's age, gender, and race are not very potent determinants. This news is gratifying confirmation that creative and competent therapists can overcome limitations potentially imposed by such arbitrary characteristics as gender, age, or skin color (Blow et al., 2007). Second, research about experience level is surprisingly mixed. Just putting in time as a therapist does not automatically increase one's expertise. Stolk and Perlesz (1990) offered data that students in the second year of a strategic marital and family therapy program actually produced worse results than did students in the first year, presumably because second-year students focused more on technique at the expense of the therapeutic alliance. Many other variables (such as the difficulty of the cases undertaken and the quality of training) probably also moderate the influence of experience on success (Beutler et al., 1998).

Therapist positivity and friendliness are consistently associated with favorable outcomes, while criticism/hostility has a negative association (Beutler et al., 2004). Therapists should manifest a sufficiently high level of activity as to interrupt clients' dysfunctional patterns, and they should also provide sufficient structure to encourage family members to face their cognitive, emotional, and behavioral issues (Bischoff & Sprenkle, 1993; Lebow, 2006b). There is evidence that therapist defensiveness, especially early in the treatment, leads to poor outcomes in couple therapy (Waldron, Turner, Barton, Alexander, & Cline, 1997).

There is consistent evidence that therapists need to adapt to client preferences, expectations, and characteristics. Beutler, Consoli, and Lane (2005) offered strong evidence that therapists should decrease directiveness (therapist control) when client resistance is high, and vice versa. Furthermore, the therapist should adjust his or her style to keep the client's emotional arousal at a moderate level (neither too high nor too low) since moderate arousal seems to facilitate change (Blow et al., 2007). Beutler, Harwood, Alimohamed, and Malik (2002) also provide impressive evidence that therapists do better offering insight-oriented procedures to clients who are more self-reflective, introspective, and introverted. Conversely, therapists should offer skill-building and symptom-focused methods to clients who are more impulsive and aggressive. There is also growing evidence that therapists whose work is sensitive to the cultural values and beliefs of clients get better results. This conclusion was supported by a review of research on poor African Americans and Hispanics in Miami by Jose Szapocznik and colleagues (Muir, Schwartz, & Szapocznic, 2004).

A more detailed summary of the findings on therapist factors in couple and family therapy and individual therapy is found in Blow and associates' work (2007). Given that, even within models, therapists vary considerably in competence, it behooves us to learn more about why, specifically, some therapists get better results. Model proponents should also want to know this information since therapists are what makes models come alive. Without therapists, models are just words on paper. Just as common factors work through models, so likewise do models work through therapists (Blow et al., 2007). Indeed, Blow et al. (2007) have stated that "it may be better to talk about empirically supported therapists than models" (p. 312).

Dimensions of the Therapeutic Relationship as Common Factors

Since Chapter 7 will focus exclusively on this topic, we will be brief here. Suffice it to say at this point that the therapeutic relationship, now studied predominantly as the multidimensional "therapeutic alliance," is the most studied common factor in couple and family therapy research. There is compelling evidence across numerous studies that this variable contributes significantly to successful outcomes in all effective models. In fact, among relational therapy models with the strongest empirical support such as emotionally focused therapy (Johnson & Denton, 2002), functional family therapy (Sexton & Alexander, 2003) and multisystemic therapy (Sheidow, Henggeler, & Schoenwald, 2003), there is a strong emphasis on building strong therapeutic alliances. The reader will recall from Chapter 3, however, that the moderate view of common factors does not posit that building strong relationships is sufficient for concluding successful therapeutic change, even though it is necessary and undoubtedly desirable.

Dimensions of Expectancy as Common Factors

In his widely cited chapter, Lambert (1992) argued that expectancy and "placebo factors" accounted for about 15% of the outcome variance in psychotherapy; again, remember that this was just a "guesstimate" on his part. These variables refer to the portion of improvement resulting from the client's knowledge of being in treatment, becoming hopeful, and believing that the treatment was credible. These variables were also an essential part of Franks's (1961) early description of common factors.

Regarding the terminology of this aspect of common factors, we prefer "expectancy" or "hope" rather than "placebo." Wampold (2001) makes the case that in medical research it is meaningful to make a distinction between the specific ingredients of a physiochemical treatment and a placebo treatment (whose impact is mostly psychological) that controls for the nonphysiochemical elements. In medicine it is feasible to deliver a purely physiochemical treatment, for example, to someone who is comatose. However, in psychotherapy the effects attributable to both specific therapeutic treatments and nonspecific alternatives are chiefly psychological. It is virtually impossible to take the nonspecific aspects out of the "specific" treatment. Lambert and Ogles (2004) point out, for example, that all treatments, including the most rigorously empirically validated ones and not just those offered to nonspecific control groups, utilize expectancy (in the sense of creating hope and credibility) to engender change. Hence, Lambert and Ogles assert—and we agree—that the term "placebo" is a misnomer.

Regarding the hope dimension, Howard, Moras, Brill, Martinovich, and Lutz (1996) argued that the beginning stage of therapy is primarily concerned with a movement from demoralization to remoralization. Although various researchers employ different terms, remoralization seems to be built into the initial stages of empirically supported relationship therapies (Sprenkle & Blow, 2004a) such as emotionally focused therapy (Johnson & Denton, 2002) and functional family therapy (Sexton & Alexander, 2003). However, there does not appear to be much research in relationship therapy specifically on the relationship between hope and change. There is some evidence regarding the credibility dimension in that several studies (Crane, Griffin, & Hill, 1986; Kuehl, Newfield, & Joanning, 1990; Johnson & Talitman, 1997) demonstrated a significant relationship between relational therapy success and the therapist's ability to offer a credible treatment that matched clients' expectations. This dimension may overlap with the "tasks" or "goals" dimensions of the therapeutic alliance (see Chapter 7).

Nonspecific Mechanisms of Change as Common Factors

This category is equivalent to the narrow view of common factors. We consider the narrow view to be a subset of the broad view. These common nonspecific mechanisms of change exist (sometimes unrecognized) in the various treatment models even though the models have different theoretical assumptions and employ techniques that look different and have different names and use different language. Despite these differences, the mechanisms achieve similar results. These mechanisms exist at a lower level of abstraction than "theories" and a higher level of abstraction than techniques (Goldfried, 1980). So, for example, solution-focused therapy and emotionally focused therapy offer different theoretical lenses for couple therapy, and they use different techniques (like the miracle question and softening, respectively); yet, at a higher level of abstraction these two techniques often both result in husbands and wives changing their views of each other from one who is hostile or distant to one who is caring. "Changing the viewing" or "altering cognitions" is the common change mechanism.

The common factors literature offers a number of lists of non-specific change mechanisms (Grencavage & Norcross, 1990; Lambert & Ogles, 2004). Since some of these lists are quite complex, we were attracted to the influential and parsimonious conceptualization offered by Karasu (1986), who said that these non-model-specific change mechanisms could be subsumed under behavioral regulation (which we also have called "changing the doing," or in Chapter 8 of this volume "altering behaviors"); cognitive mastery (which we have called "changing the viewing," or in Chapter 8 "altering cognitions"); and affective experiencing (which we have called "affective experiencing/regulation, or in Chapter 8 "experiencing emotions differently"). In Chapter 8 we will show how these three change mechanisms operate in three seemingly disparate relational couple therapies: object relations, emotionally focused, and solution-focused therapies.

We have also mentioned in this book some common mechanisms that are unique to couple and family therapy, such as conceptualizing problems systemically as dysfunctional cycles, interrupting these cycles, expanding the direct treatment system, and capitalizing on the expanded therapeutic alliance.

Other Mediating and Moderating Variables as Common Factors

It is likely that there are a number of other variables that mediate or moderate the process of change. So, this last category is something of a "catch-all" for those variables missed in the five previous categories. "Mediators" are variables that explain why and how treatments have effects. So, we could argue that "therapist competence" is a mediator that helps to explain why psychotherapy works (although we already placed this common factor in a different category). "Moderators" explain the circumstances under which treatments work or do not work. So, for example, if someone believes that including the partner in couple therapy will not work if there is currently violence in the relationship, in this instance "presence of current couple violence" moderates the effectiveness of the choice for conjoint treatment. (Using this example does not gainsay the existence of empirically supported conjoint treatment for couple violence [Stith, Rosen, & McCollum, 2002]).

Some variables can be both mediators and moderators, depending on the circumstances. In this final category within the broad view of common factors, we will discuss two more variables that help to explain the process of change, both of which mediate and moderate change. Undoubtedly, future research and theory will identify others.

Allegiance of the Therapist or the Researcher

The first is the "allegiance" of the therapist or the researcher. To what extent does the therapist or the researcher have an allegiance to the model or to the model developer (as in the case of a student of a model developer) or the person (if not the model developer) doing the research that is testing the model? These are important questions since most couple and family therapy research has been done by the developers of the models or their students. (Since allegiance is a research as well as a therapist issue, we discuss it here rather than under "therapist" variables, above; see pp. 49–53.)

Allegiance is a variable that could be either a mediator or a moderator. If, for example, treatment A looked better only because of the biases of the researcher, then research allegiance could be said to mediate the favorable result of the model. If treatment B remained an effective treatment, but lost some of its potency when it was employed by therapists with less allegiance, then we could say allegiance moderated the effectiveness of treatment B.

While having an allegiance to the model a therapist practices has benefits (see below), from a *research* perspective allegiance clouds the issue of why change is occurring. In research, when models are being compared, it clearly "stacks the deck" when one model (typically the "experimental" model) has allegiance on its side and the other (typically the "control") model does not. Obviously, if the therapists in the experimental group "truly believe" in their model and the therapists in the control group do not, the former will perform better for that reason alone. Researcher allegiance effects are probably more subtle, but something seems to happen when model developers or their students implement the experimental treatment. Their greater enthusiasm and investment, as Blow et al. (2007) put it, "unwittingly leads to a halo-type effect for the approach in the experimental condition" (p. 301). They often have procured grants to test their models and have other personal investments—like wanting to market their models—that make it hard for them to do truly unbiased research. Lest we seem judgmental, if we were doing research on common factors, our research would likely be influenced by our allegiance in ways we would not recognize.

Even if totally unintentional, these allegiance effects appear to be quite powerful. Referring to an earlier thorough investigation in which allegiance effects were coded three separate ways across a variety of studies (Luborsky et al., 1999). Luborsky et al. (2002) stated: "The correlation between the mean of 3 measures of the researcher's allegiance and the outcome of the treatments compared was a huge Pearson's r of .85 for a sample of 29 comparative treatment studies" (p. 5). This very large correlation has to make us stop and wonder just what psychotherapy research over the years has really told us! Luborsky et al. (2002) put it strongly: "This high correlation of the mean of the three allegiance measures with the outcomes of the treatments compared *implies that the usual comparison of psychotherapies has a limited validity*" (p. 5; emphasis added). Luborsky and colleagues are not alone. Wampold (2001) devotes an entire chapter in his book to allegiance effects and presents compelling empirical evidence (consistent with Luborsky et al., 2002) that allegiance effects account for much more of the outcome variance in psychotherapy than the choice of the treatment model; that is, when researchers thought they were comparing treatment models, they may unwittingly have been studying allegiance effects.

Whether one agrees with these stark conclusions or not, we do concur with Luborsky et al. (2002) that future research should include researchers from a variety of allegiances within the research team and that greater efforts need to be made to ensure that comparisons to preferred treatments are made equally credible (Sprenkle & Blow, 2004b). We believe this is particularly important for couple and family therapy research since there is very little research that is not done by the founders or their students. Graduate students of one of us (D. H. S.) examined 45 empirical articles related to three of the most widely employed relational therapy models: emotionally focused therapy, functional family therapy, and multisystemic therapy. Fewer than 10% of the published papers appear to have been done by independent investigators (Sprenkle & Blow, 2004a). Moreover, we are not aware of a single study in relationship therapy "that was a head-to-head comparison of treatments previously demonstrated to be effective, in which the study was carried out by neutral although enthusiastic experts in supportive contexts—that is, in which all treatments were equally valued (Sprenkle & Blow, 2004a, pp. 117–118).

Before closing this section on allegiance, we wish to emphasize that from a *clinical* perspective allegiance is mostly a good thing since you cannot "sell" something that you do not believe in. Allegiance can be a common factor that enhances therapy. As long as it is not "blind" allegiance that prevents therapist flexibility and sensitivity to client needs, allegiance can have a positive impact on generating hope, inspiring confidence, and appearing credible. Perhaps one of the reasons that control groups or "treatments-as-usual" are sometimes ineffective is because therapists have no allegiance to them. We can think of therapist allegiance as a mediator when it helps to explain why someone is effective. It may also function as a moderator in that some models work even better under the condition that therapists have strong allegiance to them.

Organization and Coherence of the Therapy Model

A second variable that probably mediates or moderates change is the "organization and coherence" of the therapy model, *independent* of the content of the model. We believe that one explanation for the potency of empirically validated models resides in their being very organized and coherent. The people who practice these therapies have a clear roadmap of the dysfunction they are addressing, the place where they want clients to go, and how to get there. This very organization and coherence impacts other variables we have discussed, such as the therapist's confidence and the credibility of the therapist and the model for the client.

When, say, comparing experimental treatment with a "treatment-as-usual" condition, perhaps the former is more successful not so much because of the uniqueness of the treatment but rather because it is well organized and coherent. In comparison, treatments-as-usual are sometimes carried out by well-intentioned people who are none-theless "flying by the seat of their pants." So, organization and coher-ence can be a mediator—that explains why change occurs. They could also be a moderator, in that a given treatment may work only under the condition that it is well organized and coherent.

In this chapter we have offered an overview of six aspects of the treatment setting that contribute to change within all effective models: common client, therapist, relationship (alliance), expectancy, change mechanisms, and miscellaneous mediating and moderating variables (including allegiance and the organization/coherence of a model). Since we are interactional thinkers ourselves, we want to acknowledge that these distinctions are somewhat artificial. It is hard to disentangle, for example, a common change mechanism like "alter-ing cognitions" from the therapist's belief in the mechanism, or the client's assessment of its credibility, or the client's attitude toward the person who is doing the intervention. It is also true that a variable like client motivation can be predominantly a client characteristic that he or she brings to therapy, or enhancing motivation can be seen as an aspect of being a competent therapist (Sprenkle & Blow, 2004a). Often the variables described here interact, as when a therapist uses an approach that is a good match for the strength of a client. Of course, by its very nature, the therapeutic alliance is a partnership of client and therapist. So, while we hope the six categories are heuristic, they clearly are not distinct but highly interactional. Earlier in this chap-ter we reviewed the research of Larry Beutler (Beutler et al., 2005) that tried to match principles of therapeutic treatment (like insight-oriented vs. symptom-based approaches) with type of client. There is also a school of research called "aptitude by treatment interaction" (ATI) that is based on the notion that individual clients can be matched to particular treatments tailored to the client's particular problem. The most ambitious test was in alcohol treatment (Project MATCH Research Group, 1997). However, ATI designs have been used only infrequently, and the results have been "relatively disappointing, and Project Match is a prime example" (Clarkin & Levy, 2004, p. 214). So, it will be up to future researchers to determine whether the inter-actions among variables of interest to common factors proponents can be identified in ways that will enhance treatment.

5

A Moderate View
of Common Factors

Although it sounds like an oxymoron, we are "militant moderates" when it comes to common factors. In fact, we believe that when well-intentioned advocates of common factors take an extreme position on the issue, they run the risk of giving the movement a bad name. So, at the outset of this chapter, we want to make some statements that we emphatically *don't* believe reflect our view of common factors. We clearly reject the ideas that "any one treatment is as good as any other" or "that it really doesn't matter what you do in therapy so long as you have a good relationship with your client." We also reject the notions that "treatment models are unimportant," or that "outcome research is a waste of time," or that "you have to make an either–or choice between common factors or a model-driven approach to change." One of us (D. H. S.) is fond of telling his students that the field of relationship therapy has been subjected to two major mistakes throughout its intellectual history. First, we have a tendency to "throw the baby out with the bathwater." For example, when we develop new models, we tend to ignore or denigrate classic approaches that in fact frequently form the basis for "new" approaches. Second, we have the tendency to take things to extremes. Taking a radical stance in favor of common factors is a good example.

Specifically, we propose five distinctions between the moderate and extreme positions. In so doing we wish to make clear that these two overall stances (moderate vs. extreme) are often best viewed as a continuum rather than as discrete categories. Furthermore, no authors that we know of represent the extreme position in its entirety, even though some writers, whom we otherwise admire, have made statements that could be interpreted as extreme on some dimensions. Additionally, we candidly admit that our own thinking about common factors has evolved and changed. In some of our earlier writing we ourselves took positions that we could now consider as extreme. More often than not, we hear the extreme positions voiced by people who either don't know very much about common factors or who are critical of it without knowing there is a moderate position, as articulated here. Hence, from our vantage point as "militant moderates," they are attacking a "straw man" version of common factors that we ourselves would reject. In the five distinctions that follow, the first part is the extreme view, and the second; our moderate view.

Believes One Treatment Is as Good as Another versus Questions Claims about *Relative* Efficacy

Some treatments are very efficacious, and some are not. We do not support the literal belief that any approach is just as good as another. Taken to extremes, this is a silly position since it puts an impressive empirically validated model like emotionally focused therapy (Johnson, 1996) on the same level as tarot cards, palm reading, and Ouija boards (Sprenkle & Blow, 2004a). Some treatments are quackery. For this reason, we think it is unfortunate that the term "dodo bird verdict," taken from a passage in *Alice in Wonderland* in which "everybody has won and all shall have prizes," is sometimes used as a catchphrase to describe the common factors position (Luborsky et al., 1975, 2002). It connotes the extreme position that it does not matter what you do in therapy. (Here is an example where, in our earlier writing [Sprenkle et al., 1999], at least one of us [D. H. S.] sounded more like an advocate of an extreme view since he used the catchphrase himself in that work in support of common factors.)

In contrast, our moderate common factors approach argues that among *efficacious* psychotherapies there are relatively small overall differences in treatment outcome, particularly when key confounding variables are controlled (more on this later). By "efficacious" we mean therapies that have demonstrated superiority to a control group in more than one study where there has been a randomized clinical trial (see more details at the end of this section). As we note in point 4 below, the moderate common factors position supports clinical trials research with some qualifications. The moderate common factors position is not a statement about absolute efficacy. We do not question that many models are efficacious and believe that models that have not tested their efficacy should do so. The moderate position is a statement about *relative* efficacy. As we will spell out in more detail in many parts of this book, there is very limited empirical evidence for the *relative* superiority of specific *efficacious* treatments as compared to other *efficacious* treatments. As was noted in Chapter 2, Shadish and Baldwin (2002), after reviewing all of the meta-analyses that have been completed on couple and family therapy wrote: "There is little evidence for differential efficacy among the various approaches to marriage and family interventions, particularly if mediating and moderating variables are controlled" (p. 363). Unless and until new evidence emerges, it is hard to make a strong case for the specific model-driven approach to explaining therapeutic effectiveness.

The reader may wonder about models he or she uses that have never been formally researched. In the absence of clinical trials with random assignment to treatment and control groups, we have to remain noncommital regarding whether these models are efficacious. Although there are other ways of examining efficaciousness like client surveys, nonexperimental research methods have so many threats to validity that they must be considered only secondary indicators of efficacy. As noted earlier, we advocate that model developers (better yet, independent investigators) should test not-yet-researched models for efficacy in rigorous clinical trials. However, we personally believe, based on the history of clinical trials, that if these models are based on solid social psychological principles, if they are well organized and coherent treatments that are used by large numbers of reputable clinicians, we think it is highly likely (although by no means certain) that they would prove efficacious if put to the test. As we elaborate further in Chapter 10, rarely are widely used treatments not found to be efficacious when they are formally researched with sound methods (Wampold, 2001). So, it is plainly wrong to conclude that models not yet shown to be efficacious should be assumed to be nonefficacious or worthless. Conversely, just because researchers have chosen predominantly to investigate cognitive-behavioral models, which lend themselves well to brief clinical trials, we should not assume that these approaches are necessarily superior to others (Westen, Novotny, & Thompson-Brenner, 2004). After all, as we note numerous times in this volume, in the most expensive and arguably the most unbiased outcome study ever completed, the NIH Collaborative Study of

Depression, a brief psychodynamic model performed just as well as cognitive-behavioral therapy (Blatt et al., 1996).

Regarding what constitutes an "efficacious" treatment, we offer two additional observations. First, let us note something about terminology. Pinsof and Wynne (1995), in their review of outcome research in marriage and family therapy, stressed the important distinction between "efficacy" and "effectiveness" research. They noted the vast majority of the studies in relational therapy have measured "efficacy" since they were done in controlled settings removed from the realities of typical clinical practice. In efficacy research there is more emphasis on "internal" validity (that is, proving that the experimental treatment is what causes the result). Research done in more real-world contexts is called "effectiveness" research, and it focuses more on external validity (showing that the results of the study generalize to other settings). More recently, Shadish and Baldwin (2002) have confirmed that there is still insufficient evidence to say with certainty whether most relational interventions work well under the conditions of actual clinical practice. There are just not enough clinically representative studies. The two terms ("efficacy" and "effectiveness"), however, while sometimes distinguished in the literature along the lines of Pinsof and Wynne (1995), are also widely used interchangeably. For example, the book *Effectiveness Research in Marriage and Family Therapy* (Sprenkle, 2002) is really mostly about efficacy studies. In the literature, treatments are often called "effective" when they should be more accurately labeled "efficacious." Writers sometimes avoid the latter term because it seems more cumbersome and more technical. In this book, when we slip into the more vernacular term "effective," the reader should understand we would be more technically correct if we said "efficacious."

Our second detail concerns the scientific debate regarding how efficacy is established within the clinical trials framework. We tend to agree with Shadish and Baldwin (2002), themselves proponents of clinical trials research and rigorous methods, that the widely cited standards set by Division 12 of the American Psychological Association (Chambless & Hollon, 1998) are too restrictive. To become an empirically supported treatment, not only must a method achieve results superior to a control group in two investigations, but also the method must be targeted to a specific population and specified in a treatment manual. Shadish and Baldwin (2002) argue that this definition marginalizes many therapies that are well supported through meta-analysis but do not have treatment manuals or have not specified target populations to the extent the EST definitions require. They believe that, as they are currently defined, ESTs are really just one type of empirically supported treatment and might be more accurately labeled "effective, manualized, population specific" treatments (Shadish & Baldwin, 2002, p. 350). They argue that a variety of other treatments have received recognition from governments and scholarly bodies that do not meet today's criteria for an EST. Shadish and Baldwin propose what they call "meta-analytically supported" treatments, or MASTS. To be designated a MAST would require that the approach be the subject of a meta-analysis (minimum of two studies) and that the studies in the meta-analysis be randomized trials comparing the treatment to a control group. Shadish and Baldwin report that, while only 5 couple and family therapies meet the requirement for being an EST, 24 meet the criteria for a MAST, including such broad categories as systemic marital therapy and systemic family therapy. We support Shadish and Baldwin's broader definition for what it should mean to be an empirically supported treatment.

To summarize this section, the moderate view of common factors does not suggest that just "any approach" will do. The approach should be *efficacious*. But what we do challenge is that there is much evidence for *relative* efficacy among those methods shown to be efficacious.

Disparages Effective Models versus Supports Them

Psychotherapy models are usually a good thing—in fact, they are probably needed for therapists to do their work effectively. However, as with the preceding discussion, not all models are equally good. At some level there could also be a "model" behind the use of tarot cards or Ouija boards in therapy. So, models are probably inevitable since all therapists have a repetitive pattern in the work that they do, but that does not mean that the model necessarily focuses on relevant data or is helpful. It may simply be preaching what Aunt Martha thinks makes a good relationship. So, not all models are necessarily effective, and when we say we support models we mean models that either have been demonstrated to be effective or at least incorporate social psychological principles that have been shown to be useful and helpful in the scientific literature. (A fair number of couple and family therapies, including, for example, most of the intergenerational and older experiential models—contemporary emotionally focused therapy [Johnson, 1996] is a notable exception—have very little formal outcome research to back them up. Nevertheless, they are coherent, plausible models rooted in valid social psychological principles.)

The moderate common factors position does not take issue with models per se (that is, effective or plausible ones) but only with the issue of *why* they work. We take the position that effective models are *mostly* effective because they do a credible job of activating or potentiating the common factors that are primarily responsible for therapeutic change.

Common factors are not "islands," but rather they work through models (Sprenkle & Blow, 2004b). To change the metaphor, if common factors drive change, then models are the roadmaps therapists use to get where they are going. A therapist is bombarded with 10,000 bits of information a second (Watzlawick, Beavin, & Jackson, 1967). If for no other reason, models are needed for the therapist to filter the information most relevant for successful treatment of the client. Furthermore, models give the therapist a conceptual map of what is dysfunctional about the current situation as well as what would be a more functional alternative. To a large extent, therapy is about the process of helping clients get from a not-so-good point *A* to a better or much better point *B*. Models also afford clients credible roadmaps regarding the issues for which they come to therapy and viable alternative routes to a better life. We support models since common factors work through them; and, as noted below, you have to do "something" in therapy beyond developing a caring relationship. Our only issue is with model proponents who claim that their models work largely through mechanisms that are unique or distinctive. We believe what they share with other effective models accounts for most of their curative attributes.

Sees the Therapeutic Relationship as All There Is versus Views the Relationship as Only One Aspect of Change

A very common misinterpretation of common factors is that they are *all* about the therapeutic relationship or therapeutic alliance. In this view, models mean little and the therapeutic relationship means everything. Indeed, some scholars (Patterson, 1984) have argued that the therapeutic relationship is not only necessary to therapeutic change but is actually *sufficient*—in other words, that having a good therapeutic alliance is all that is necessary for change to occur. Although we do believe that the therapeutic relationship is a highly significant factor in treatment outcome and certainly necessary for change to occur, our position is that a much larger array of common factors must also be present to explain change. Suffice it to say this is another aspect of our belief that you have "do something" in therapy besides relate well to clients (Sprenkle & Blow, 2004a). Although important, the alliance is only one aspect of helping clients solve their problems.

Minimizes Clinical Trials Research versus Supports It

Some proponents of common factors whose opinions we otherwise respect greatly (Duncan & Miller, 2000; Wampold, 2001) take a dimmer view of clinical trials research than we do (Sprenkle & Blow, 2004a). As we noted earlier, useful models must be proven efficacious, and randomized clinical trials are the only method respected by external audiences like third-party payers and government agencies to demonstrate such efficaciousness or effectiveness. We think it is extremely important that couple and family therapies get this kind of validation. Furthermore, as we develop further in Chapter 10, secondary evidence (through meta-analysis) of clinical trials research is the basis for a large part of the evidence for the common factors paradigm.

We also believe that, although many common factors cannot be experimentally manipulated (see Chapter 10 for more details), there is nothing inherent in the methodology of clinical trials that would prevent many common factors from being investigated. Unfortunately, clinical trials to date have been predicated on the assumption that what distinguishes successful from unsuccessful outcomes is the particular model being tested—to the exclusion of other sources of variance. (For example, there are important therapist variables independent of the model that the therapist is using; even well-trained therapists employing the same model often get dramatically different results [Blatt et al., 1996]). However, differential therapist results and other variables related to common factors (like the allegiance of the therapist to the model) can be incorporated into the methodology for randomized clinical trials. We also strongly believe that common factors should be investigated through other methods like process research and qualitative research. However, our purpose here is to stress that throwing out the "gold standard" of randomized clinical trials may be "throwing the baby out with the bathwater."

Supports Either–Or versus Both–And
in the Common Factors and Specific Factors Debate

We also reject taking a "hard line" in the common factors versus specific factors debate. Although we contrasted the model-driven and common-factors-driven paradigms of change in Chapter 1, we stressed that the two are not polar opposites but rather something in between. In individual therapy, for example, there is reasonable evidence that for certain specific problems, like the treatment of phobias, panic disorder, and compulsions, behavioral (Emmelkamp, 2004) and cognitive methods (Hollon & Beck, 2004) appear to offer added benefit that cannot be explained away by the kind of mediating and moderating variables that so often make outcome research more biased than meets the eye. As we noted in Chapter 4 and will reinforce with more details in Chapter 10, some clinical trials compare a well-organized and coherent approach, enthusiastically endorsed by the therapists, with a disorganized and noncoherent approach to which therapists have little allegiance. Rarely is the control group as credible as what the best clinicians in private practice are doing to treat the problem (Westen et al., 2004). When the deck is stacked in this way, it is not clear that the specific unique aspects of the experimental treatment are what differentiate it from the control group. However, in our judgment the research is compelling enough around some specific problems (phobias, panic disorder, and compulsions) that we think treatment specificity clearly adds something important.

Our main point here is that we are open to the possibility that some specific treatments add to the common factors that underlie all effective treatments. We consider ourselves "evidence people," and whenever there is methodologically sound and unbiased evidence for specificity, we are pleased to embrace it. As Carl Rogers said, "The facts are always friendly" (cited in Asay & Lambert, 1999, p. 49).

We also think that, within the realm of couple and family therapy, certain general types or classes of therapy are probably more effective for certain problems. For example, it is probably the case that working with conduct-disordered adolescents requires approaches that are ecologically based, highly structured, and quite active. Relational therapy has four very effective approaches to working with this population, including functional family therapy (Sexton & Alexander, 2003), multisystemic therapy (Sheidow et al., 2003), brief strategic family therapy (Szapocznik & Williams, 2000), and multidimensional family therapy (Liddle et al., 2002). There is little evidence, however, that they are *differentially* effective—relative to one another. So, the general type of therapy may make a specific difference, even though the specific models within this general type of therapy may not be more or less effective than one another. There is also some strong evidence, as we mentioned in Chapter 3, that there is a "unit-of-treatment" effect for certain problems. The reader may recall the list of problems for which using conjoint versus individual units of treatment appears to be additive. We believe these differences are real and not methodological artifacts. Again, when there is compelling evidence, we are open to qualifying the common factors hypothesis.

Having taken the both–and position, we still believe it is highly likely that future research will still demonstrate that common factors account for considerably more of the outcome variance in psychotherapy than specific factors. Furthermore, we also believe that the enthusiastic proponents of certain models need to be more modest and to give common factors more credit. Nonetheless, if credible evidence were to shift the balance more in the direction of specific factors, we would "go with the evidence."

Table 5.1 summarizes the end points on the five continua we have described, comparing the extreme versus moderate positions on common factors.

TABLE 5.1. Extreme versus Moderate Position on Common Factors

Extreme position	Moderate position
Believes one treatment is as good as another.	Questions relative efficacy of treatments, but considers absolute efficacy important.
Disparages models.	Affirms models are important as the vehicles through which common factors operate.
Asserts the therapeutic relationship is everything.	Says that, while important, the therapeutic relationship is only one aspect of helping clients.
Devalues clinical trials.	Values clinical trials but also encourages their use in studying common factors when feasible.
Takes an "either–or" stance.	Values "both–and" in the debate on common factors versus specific factors.

6

Getting Clients Fired Up
for a Change

Matching Therapist Behavior
with Client Motivation

Clients as the Most Important Common Factor

We always find it interesting to find out what "outsiders" think about our profession. One of us (S. D. D.) was recently at a party with several nontherapist friends when one of them asked what I researched and wrote about the most. Realizing that the party was about to take a turn for the worse, I nevertheless launched into a plain English explanation of common factors. "Well, wouldn't the client be the most important part of therapy?" a friend asked. "A lot of people are starting to think so," I replied. "Starting to think so?" he said. "That seems pretty obvious to me! I mean, if you want to change, you're going to change, unless maybe your therapist is a jerk or something, but then you could just go somewhere else." The rest of my friends looked at me like they wanted to say, with incredulity, "Your field *just* started arriving at that conclusion? I could have told you that!" but they kindly refrained and the conversation drifted into something more interesting.

My friends had a good point. I remember vividly (with a grin now, but it was very humbling at the time!) an instance in which I was working with an adult client who was struggling with the effects of childhood abuse. Midway through one of our sessions I launched into some brilliant (or so I thought) explanation of a concept I thought related to her situation. I was really humming along; I was even sur-

69

prising myself with my insights! My client waited patiently until I fin-
ished, at which point I asked her what she thought about what I had
said. I was confident that she would be changed in some way. "Honestly?" she asked. "Of course," I replied. "I wouldn't have it any
other way." "Whaah, whaah, whaah," she said, imitating the voice
on the Snoopy cartoon! "I honestly didn't understand a word you
said, but while you were talking I started thinking about something
else," and she went on to mention a new insight that she had into her
problem, and actions she was going to take as a result of her insight.
Needless to say, I felt pretty sheepish. Seemingly the main benefit that
I had given her with my insights was time for her to think while I
talked! This was a watershed experience for me, though, as I realized
that clients are often more resourceful than we give them credit for.
They take what we give them and make it work, sometimes in spite
of our best efforts! Like my friends at the party said, it is strange that
the centrality of the client has become of interest mostly in the past
decade or so.

    Many of the ensuing clinical chapters in this book focus on com-
monalities across relational therapy theories. This is what we described
in Chapter 1 as the *narrow* view of common factors. We will emphasize these common change processes because we believe such a discussion is absent in the relational therapy literature and because we
think identifying relationships between core relational therapy processes and interventions can greatly simplify practice, research, and
training. However, it is a common mistake when reading between the
lines of chapters that focus on techniques—common or otherwise—
to assume that it is what the *therapist* does that is the most important element of therapy. Therefore, we wanted to begin the clinical
chapters by reiterating the importance of clients (as we discussed in
Chapter 5) for one reason: we believe, as do many common factors
researchers, that it is in fact *clients* that are the most important common factor in the success or failure of therapy (Duncan & Miller,
2000). Recall, as we pointed out in Chapter 1, that a broad (versus a
narrow) view of common factors includes all aspects of the treatment
setting that contribute to change, and clients are the ones that take
diverse approaches and fashion them to suit their needs. Clients are
the ones who choose what to pay attention to and how to make it
work. Tallman and Bohart (1999) express it well:

    Therapy facilitates naturally occurring healing aspects of clients'
    lives. Therapists function as support systems and resource provid-

ers. This view contrasts with most of the literature on psychotherapy. There, the therapist is the "hero" who, with potent techniques and procedures, intervenes in clients' lives and fixes their malfunctioning machinery, be they faulty cognitions, weak and ineffectual egos, primitive defensive structures, conditioned maladaptive behaviors, defective social skills, or poorly working internal self-organizations. (p. 91)

One message implicit in the countless hours spent learning therapy, attending workshops, and so forth is that the success or failure of therapy is riding on the therapists' shoulders. Perhaps another reason for the traditional view is that clients do not typically write therapy training manuals or give engaging presentations at therapy conferences highlighting the magic of what they do, so we are left to believe that it is indeed therapists who are responsible for most of the change in therapy. Invoking the contrary view, this chapter will focus on conducting model-informed therapy in a manner that works *with* clients' self-healing capacity rather than *against* it (e.g., by doing therapy "to" or "on" clients, much as they would have surgery done "to" or "on" them).

That said, our moderate common factors paradigm differs from that of other common factors researchers in that we favor a more balanced view of client and therapist factors. Therapists *do* matter; a poor therapist may thwart even the most motivated client, and a good therapist may be able to motivate a client with low motivation. Although we believe that client variables are the most important factor in therapy, we worry that common factors researchers sometimes take this emphasis to the extreme. An overemphasis on client factors can have several damaging effects. Overemphasizing client factors may unduly discourage a therapist, leading him or her to think that nothing he or she might do would make a difference anyway—so, why try? Similarly, it could encourage therapist laziness and a lack of a sense of accountability to clients.

When we talk about the "client" or the "therapist" as common factors, we are talking about related and reciprocal dimensions of the process of change; they are not unrelated entities. Although engaged and motivated clients are essential to change, what therapists do or do not do in therapy has an impact on the extent to which clients become engaged in the process. The client's engagement, in turn, has an impact on the therapist's motivation and behavior.

Mike had just told his wife Julie that he slept with a coworker on a recent business trip, and Julie insisted that Mike attend therapy to save the marriage. Mike agreed, and they called Luis in a panic to arrange a first session. The next day Julie told Luis that she knew their marriage had been bad for a long time and that this was a "huge wake-up call" for her to take Mike's complaints about the relationship seriously. Mike felt awful about what he had done and also expressed a strong desire to work on the marriage. Some friends had recently endured an affair, and they assured Mike and Julie that their marriage was stronger because they stuck together.

Unbeknown to Mike and Julie, Luis had left his wife the year before because of her infidelity, and he was still going through his own healing on the issue. Overwhelmed by their all-too-familiar emotions, he ignored their expressed wishes and recommended that Mike and Julie separate for a few months to clear their heads and make sure they wanted to continue the marriage. Stunned and confused by this line of advice, Mike and Julie reluctantly returned to Luis's office for three more sessions. Luis used these sessions to emphasize and elaborate on the problems in their marriage, and he urged them to consider whether they really wanted to remain together. Fortunately, Mike and Julie decided to fire Luis before they lost all hope, and their next therapist helped them to rebuild what hope remained and work through the affair.

In sum, we believe that client motivation is one of the—if not *the*—most important variables in therapy, but therapists can do a great deal to influence client motivation, for better or worse. Matching therapist behavior with client motivation, therefore, becomes one of the most paramount tasks of any therapeutic approach. The purpose of this chapter is to discuss how therapists can match their behavior with their clients' level of motivation to help them become more motivated and engaged in therapy. To these ends, we will review two different meta-theories, namely, Prochaska's transtheoretical stages-of-change model (Prochaska, 1999) and Miller and Rollnick's motivational interviewing (2002). Even though these models were developed to explain motivation and change in substance abuse approaches for individuals, many principles apply for motivating entire systems as well. Nevertheless, motivating an entire system requires additional skills. We use functional family therapy (Sexton & Alexander, 2003) as an example of a systemic model that recognizes the importance of client motivation and incorporates motivational interviewing and transtheoretical stages-of-change principles into the model. There are a number of couple and family therapy models that also overlap with principles of client engagement and motivation as outlined by

Prochaska (1999) and Miller and Rollnick (2002). We will end with a clinical case vignette illustrating how principles from each of the three models interact to produce change in a family system.

Transtheoretical Stages-of-Change Model

Prochaska and colleagues (Prochaska, DiClemente, & Norcross, 1992) believe that all clients are motivated, although client motivation looks very different, depending on which "stage of change" the client is in. Instead of clients being unmotivated, resistant, and so forth, rather they are *differently* motivated. Prochaska and colleagues (1992) found that when people change they cycle through six distinct stages several times before permanently changing a behavior. Since different goals and interventions (Prochaska and colleagues call them "processes of change"; 1992, p. 1107) are better suited for different stages, it becomes the therapist's task to match the two: "Efficient self-change depends on doing the right things (processes) at the right times (stages)" (p. 1110). Since different therapy models emphasize different processes of change (e.g., psychodynamic insight vs. behavioral action), the question is not "which model is the best" but rather "which model utilizes processes of change best suited for this client's current stage of change?" (As an aside, the ability to match model-specific interventions to a client's current stage of change presupposes that therapists are competent in several different models, one of the cornerstone claims of our moderate common factors approach. We provide guidance for mastering several different models in Chapter 11.)

The Stages and Processes of Change

The six stages of change are precontemplation, contemplation, preparation, action, maintenance, and termination. It is important to note that people rarely progress through each stage in a linear manner. Rather, people often fall back to earlier stages, learning through each regression and doing better the next time around (Prochaska et al., 1992). The nine processes of change are consciousness raising, dramatic relief, environmental reevaluation, self-reevaluation, self-liberation, contingency management, helping relationships, counterconditioning, and stimulus control (Prochaska, 1999). We will review each stage of change and the processes of change most closely associated with that stage.

Precontemplation

Clients in the precontemplation stage are not intending to change anytime in "the next 6 months" (Prochaska, 1999, p. 228). They are either unaware of or underinformed about the severity of their problem. Even if they think they have a problem, they view the costs of change as far outweighing any of the benefits. If they end up in treatment, it is often at the behest of significant others in their life or the legal system. If they do arrive in treatment, they are often labeled as "resistant." People can remain in the precontemplation stage for years.

Devon and Stevonea thought it was normal for Devon to storm out of the house when he was angry with Stevonea. He would often stay away for days, spending most of his time socializing with his friends. When he came home, the couple would remain silent for a while and then return to a tense truce until the next fight. Stevonea rarely if ever told Devon what she really felt. This pattern had always existed; they had each seen it in their parents and grandparents for as long as they could remember.

For clients to move from precontemplation to contemplation, they need to increase the number of "pros" (vs. "cons") they see in a life without the problem (Prochaska, 1994). Therefore, clinical efforts in this stage should focus on increasing insight. *Consciousness-raising* processes of change are well suited for this stage. Examples of this might include bibliotherapy, psychoeducation, making lists of the positive consequences of changing, envisioning a life without the problem, and so on. *Dramatic relief* processes of change that focus on arousing emotions related to the problem are helpful at this stage as well. Such interventions can include role plays, envisioning life later if the problem persists, and experiential interventions. *Environmental reevaluation* processes of change are the third group of interventions that are useful with those in the precontemplation stage. These interventions include having family members describe how they perceive the client, helping the client gain empathy for those in his or her environment that are impacted by his or her behavior, and so forth (Prochaska, 1999).

Contemplation

In this stage, clients anticipate taking action "in the next 6 months" (Prochaska, 1999, p. 229). They are unhappy with their problem and want to be rid of it, but they are also very much aware of the reasons not to change. They will often vacillate between getting angry about their problem and indulging in it. This stage is often considered "chronic contemplation or behavioral procrastination" (Prochaska, 1999, p. 230).

Devon and Stevonea were having a barbecue with their new neighbors, Kevin and Almesha, when suddenly Kevin and Almesha got into an argument. Devon and Stevonea were surprised to see that, even though things got pretty heated between them, neither one bolted from the scene, both preferring to confront each other directly throughout the argument. Devon and Stevonea even saw Kevin and Almesha quietly walking hand in hand later that evening. For a while, Devon thought that Kevin must be a wimp, and Stevonea thought that Almesha needed to "learn her place" in the home. Despite these judgments, Kevin and Almesha found themselves spending more and more time with their neighbors simply because it "felt good" in their house. After a while, Stevonea started noticing that Devon no longer immediately rushed out the door whenever they began to argue.

From time to time, Kevin and Almesha good-naturedly encouraged Devon and Stevonea to go to couple counseling. At first they did not want to, but as the months wore on Devon and Stevonea had to admit that they had never seen a marriage as happy as Kevin and Almesha's, and they agreed to a trial session. To Devon and Stevonea's relief, Lisa, the therapist, listened to what each had to say; Devon was surprised when the therapist did not get upset when Devon told her that he thought therapy was "for wimps." Both liked the fact that Lisa did not push her own agenda but rather helped them explore what they wanted from therapy since they were not sure themselves, beyond "what Kevin and Almesha had." Lisa once asked about Devon's habit of running away during a fight, and Stevonea's tendency to not share her feelings, but each became defensive. In response, Lisa left it alone for a time.

People in the contemplation stage are not very good candidates for behaviorally focused, action-oriented programs. Their motivation is not yet at the level where they will put all of their heart into behavioral change efforts. Rather, they are better-suited for more passive insight-oriented approaches that help them explore their problem, weigh the pros and cons of changing, and so forth. People in this stage have to decrease the cons of changing in order to move to action (Prochaska, Velicer, & Rossi, 1994). Therefore, the same three processes of change recommended for those in the precontemplation stage are recommended for the contemplation stage. Additionally, *self-reevaluation* processes of change are recommended as a means of moving from contemplation to preparation. Whereas environmental reevaluation focuses on the client's external environment, self-reevaluation focuses on how the client sees him- or herself with and without the problem. Interventions such as guided imagery, values clarification, encouraging congruence between one's values and behaviors, and the like can be helpful in this stage (Prochaska, 1999).

Preparation

Clients in the preparation stage are making significant plans to take action within about a month. People in the preparation stage are ready to make use of active, behavioral change-focused interventions (Prochaska, 1999).

One time Devon returned home a few hours after an argument rather visibly shaken. He'd been in a car accident, and a friend who was also in the car was in serious condition at the hospital. Something about seeing his friend and grieving wife at the hospital had made Devon rethink the way he had been treating Stevonea. Stevonea welcomed this change of attitude, as she had reached new conclusions about her own enabling behavior recently by talking with Almesha. Later that week in counseling Devon mentioned this incident, and Lisa asked what specific things Devon and Stevonea would like to change. With Lisa's guidance, the conversation gradually moved to Devon's habit of running away from—and Stevonea's stoic silence during—their altercations, and Lisa explored this pattern of interaction with them. Lisa also helped them to explore and begin practicing alternative methods of arguing.

In order to progress from preparation to action, clients must increase the "pros" of changing twice as much as they decrease their "cons" for changing (Prochaska, 1994). Therefore, self-reevaluation, with its focus on the positive aspects of life without the problem, is still an ideal process of change in this stage. *Self-liberation* is another process of change that helps clients transition to the action stage. Helpful interventions may include public commitments to work on the problem, therapist and other testaments to the client's ability to change, and the like.

Action

In this stage, people have made overt, measurable, and clinically significant changes in their life within the past six months. Ideally, people will recover during the action stage. Like those in the preparation stage, people in this stage are well suited for action-oriented approaches to change. Clients in this stage will likely get frustrated with insight-oriented approaches—they have already done that work. People work especially hard during this stage, shoring up their defenses against relapse, learning new skills and techniques, and so forth.

At first, Devon and Stevonea did not do very well with their new ways of communicating, but through diligent effort in therapy they were soon able to consistently break with their previous destructive cycle of interaction. Lisa helped them by closely examining the emotions underlying their customary behavior, exploring the cultural and gender influences on their behavior, and practicing new ways of communicating with them. Though the going was tough, they stuck with the treatment.

Self-liberation is still an effective area of work during the early phases of the action stage, as it can continue to bolster the client's confidence that he or she will succeed at changing. However, once the client is fully motivated to change, that motivation is best sustained by giving it a clear path. Thus, active behaviorally focused interventions work especially well in this stage. Therapists help clients learn to replace old behaviors with healthier alternatives. Relaxation techniques, stress management, communication skills training, and cognitive self-talk are all examples of interventions used at this stage. *Contingency management* is another process of change in which people are encouraged to set up rewards and punishments for taking steps in certain directions. Rewards for progress are generally more effective than punishments for failing (Prochaska, 1999). Social reinforcement (e.g., having a spouse thank their partner for healthy behavior) can be helpful in the short term, but self-reinforcement is generally better for the long-term maintenance of change (Prochaska et al., 1992). *Stimulus control* is another process of change in which "triggers" of past problem behaviors are avoided, changed, or otherwise removed from one's life. *Helping relationships* are the final process of change in the action stage. Clients maintain change by eliciting the help of those around them, whether therapists, family members, support groups, or others.

Maintenance

As the name of this stage suggests, change continues and a special effort is placed on whatever is needed to maintain and consolidate gains. As a natural consequence of the action stage, clients in the maintenance stage have learned from their successes and thus "are less tempted to relapse and increasingly more confident that they can continue their changes" (Prochaska, 1999, p. 231). Therapists often best help clients in the maintenance stage by helping them anticipate and prepare for challenges as well as celebrating the progress already made.

Devon and Stevonea started experiencing the episodes of their typical fighting behavior less and less frequently. When they did experience an episode, they were able to recover from it more quickly than before, thanks in part to the fact that they had practiced alternative approaches so much in therapy. Over time, reported successes in avoiding their previous interactional patterns outside of therapy enabled them to relate to each other much better.

Termination

In this stage, "individuals experience zero temptation and 100% self-efficacy" (Prochaska, 1999, p. 232). They no longer worry about a return to old behaviors because they no longer experience any temptation to do so. This is true regardless of whether or not they are exposed to old "triggers" of the problem behavior. Research suggests that, of former smokers and alcoholics, less than 20% reach this stage (Snow, Prochaska, & Rossi, 1992).

After 6 months, Devon and Stevonea were consistently able to relate to each other honestly through an argument without Devon running away and Stevonea retreating into passivity. Their marital satisfaction was greater than it had ever been. They terminated therapy, with Lisa's encouragement and assurance that they could always resume treatment if the need ever arose.

Facilitating Client Engagement through Motivational Interviewing

Like the stages-of-change model, the motivational interviewing approach (Miller & Rollnick, 2002) contends that there is no such thing as an unmotivated client—there are only therapists that are out of sync with a client's motivation. Though motivational interviewing was also developed primarily for substance-abusing clients, we believe that similar principles apply for systemic therapy. We believe that there is no such thing as an unmotivated client system, though there may be clients that have more invested in the system's current homeostasis than others. Similar to the motivational interviewing therapist's job of gently leading the substance abusing client to a life free of substances, the systemic therapist's job is to guide the system to a new homeostasis by aligning with each member's level of motivation. Motivational interviewing blends nicely with the stages-of-change model (Prochaska et al., 1992), as it provides concrete guidance for leading people through the stages of change. Miller (1995), a founder of motivational interviewing, says that "understanding the [stages] of change can help the [motivational interviewing] therapist to empathize with the client, and give direction to intervention strategies" (p. 3). Motivational interviewing offers the following five principles to get in sync with a client's motivation and help lead him or her toward change: (1) express empathy, (2) develop discrepancy, (3) avoid argumentation, (4) roll with the resistance, and (5) support self-efficacy (Miller & Rollnick, 2002). These five principles guide therapy through the following three broad stages: (1) building motivation for change, (2) strengthening commitment to change, and (3) the follow-through. There are several interventions for each stage, based on the basic principles of motivational interviewing.

Like the stance urged by many systemic approaches, a motivational interviewing therapist is kind, empathetic, and not forceful. Although there are several techniques that a therapist can use in each stage of therapy (it is a manualized treatment), emphasis is placed on getting the "spirit" of the principles of the approach as much as mastering the techniques. The therapist focuses on joining with clients in much the same way that a horse whisperer "joins up" with his or her horse (Miller, 2000): (1) by letting the person know that his or her agency is respected and the person will not be forced to change; (2) by standing still and yet inviting closeness at the same time; (3) by going with (instead of against) whatever resistance is encountered; and (4) once trust is established, by gently leading the person to health at his or her own pace.

Expressing empathy is the first principle that guides this approach. The client's freedom of choice and agency are respected; the client is viewed as the only person who can decide to change. Respect for this agency is communicated through *listening* rather than *telling* (Miller, 1995). The therapist is more of a "supportive companion and knowledge consultant" (p. 4) than a forceful instigator of change.

Developing discrepancy is the second principle of change in motivational interviewing. "Motivation for change occurs when people *perceive a discrepancy between where they are and where they want to be"* (Miller, 1995, p. 4; emphasis in original). Depending on which stage of change the client is in, the therapist focuses on gently amplifying the discrepancy that is already there (for those in the contemplation or preparation stages) or developing a discrepancy (for those in the precontemplation stage).

Avoiding argumentation is another key principle of motivational interviewing, as efforts to develop discrepancy can lead to defensiveness if not undertaken properly. Clients are not expected to admit a problem or diagnosis (e.g., "I'm an addict"). Arguments from the client are seen as evidence that the therapist does not understand the client: the therapist is going *against*, rather than *with*, the client. "When [motivational interviewing] is conducted properly, *it is the client and not the therapist that voices the arguments for change"* (Miller, 1995, p. 5; emphasis in original). This principle can be very challenging for a systemic therapist working with a client who is abusing his wife, for example. In this case, the therapist can clearly outline the husband's responsibility for the abuse but must do so in a way that validates and empowers the wife yet minimizes the husband's defensiveness while maintaining his dignity.

Rolling with the resistance is a hallmark of the motivational interviewing approach (Miller & Rollnick, 2002). Wherever the client is at the time is viewed as okay and is explored with the therapist. Ambivalence, anger, lack of motivation—they are all explored and validated rather than challenged. As the therapist rolls with the resistance, resistance often melts away, and the client comes up with his or her own solutions to the problem. Since motivational interviewing deliberately does not define what a client "should" be doing or have any specific techniques to get a client to a place the therapist determines as important (e.g., learning healthy cognitions, etc.), the therapist does not get into a power struggle with the client. The motivational interviewing therapist trusts that, given the right environment, the client will think of his or her own solutions to the problem and, since the client "owns" the solution, will be much more likely to effectuate it.

Supporting self-efficacy—the belief that one *can* change—is the fifth motivational interviewing principle of change. Unless a person believes that he or she can change, "a discrepancy crisis is likely to resolve into defensive coping (e.g., rationalization, denial) to reduce discomfort, without changing behavior" (Miller, 1995, p. 5).

The two models discussed so far were developed largely to help motivate individual substance abusers, although the stages-of-change model has since been extended to several other conditions (Prochaska,

1994). Nevertheless, both models are focused on the individual client rather than the client and his or her systems. Despite this proviso, many systemic models use similar principles to motivate clients, although the added people in the room require some differences in approach.

Facilitating Client Engagement and Motivation in Relational Therapy: Functional Family Therapy

Functional family therapy is one example of many well-defined systemic family therapy models with a clear framework and set of techniques for instilling hope (Sexton & Alexander, 2003). Like motivational interviewing, functional family therapists do not simply meet with a family and start telling them what to do; they watch the family carefully to determine family members' level of "resistance" and adjust their style and interventions accordingly. Also, as with motivational interviewing, the first and most important phase of functional family therapy is engagement and motivation. The goals associated with the engagement phase are to (1) reduce negativity and blaming, (2) redefine problems with a family focus, and (3) create a balanced therapeutic alliance.

Anyone on the receiving end of blame from the therapist or others in treatment will likely become defensive and lose motivation to participate in treatment (Onedera, 2006). Unfortunately, distressed family members often blame one another for their problems, creating a complicated web of blame that can suck the life out of a family. Many therapists unwittingly fall into this trap, assigning blame to one person (e.g., Dad's drinking) or something outside the family (e.g., a bad neighborhood). Members of these families often enter treatment in a defensive posture and ready to accuse one another. If a family comes in for treatment and the therapist asks what is wrong, family members will immediately start blaming one another for their problems, and motivation can quickly slip away. The problem with assigning blame is that those family members who are not blamed feel excused from working on the problem—the son who refuses to stop acting out because Dad's drinking is the problem; the parents who do not learn parenting skills because their son's attention-deficit/hyperactivity disorder is the problem. In functional family therapy, negativity and blaming are reduced by *reframing* what the family believes are individual problems (e.g., Johnny's acting out) as complicated family problems with no one person to blame for their occurrence. Negative relational themes that are established as problems are *reframed* with a positive focus; for example, Mom's controlling becomes her efforts to show her concern or fear for her children's safety, and so forth.

As a functional family therapist focuses on being respectful, listening to each family member, reducing negativity and blaming, and reframing problems with a family focus, the therapeutic alliance begins to form. The family begins to feel relief from its problems and feels hope that things can change. Sexton and Alexander (2003) have the following to say about the motivating effects of the alliance:

> Therapeutic motivation (an incentive to change or to act) [is] a relational process (alliance) that is an early therapeutic goal that is based on the alliance (a relational process). In FFT, motivation has an intrapersonal (within the client), a family interpersonal (between family members), and a therapeutic (between the therapist and each family member) component. When activated in a therapeutic way, each of these components contributes to producing an incentive to action. (p. 333)

The first stages of functional family therapy are very similar in conceptualization and intervention to the precontemplation and contemplation stages of Prochaska's stages-of-change model (Pochaska et al., 1992) and require very similar interventions in spirit to motivational interviewing (Miller & Rollnick, 2002). It is also very similar to the first stage of the couple therapy common factors model presented in Chapter 9. All view the therapeutic alliance as essential for motivation, and all form the alliance by not overtly trying to get clients to stop or start some behavior (e.g., stop abusing drugs, start going to school), because such an approach increases blame and reduces motivation. Rather, each model builds the alliance through a more respectful, complementary approach in which clients are listened to, problems are validated and reframed as being larger than one person, and resistance is "rolled with." As this happens, clients stop fighting themselves, one another, and the therapist to engage with treatment—not because they have been forced to but because they sincerely believe that there is hope!

Applying Principles of Motivation to Relational Therapy: A Clinical Vignette

The transtheoretical model has been applied to health engendering behaviors (e.g., diet, exercise, mammograms), compulsive behaviors (e.g., sex, food, gambling), the management of chronic health conditions, and the management of organizational change, to name a few (Prochaska, 1999). The motivational interviewing approach has been applied primarily to substance abuse (Miller, 1995). We are unaware of any application of the stages-of-change or motivational interviewing models to couple and family therapy. We will provide a brief example of how principles from these models may be used in couple and family therapy.

The Adamson family consisted of the father, Roger; the mother, Maggie; the 17-year-old son, Frank; the 14-year-old son, Ed; and a 12-year-old daughter, Melissa. They presented for therapy over concerns related to Frank's "acting out and recent run-in with the law." Roger and Maggie (especially Roger) wanted to know why Frank could not "behave like Ed and Melissa." Ed and Melissa were very quiet and reserved, rarely if ever getting into trouble. Frank, on the other hand, was a little more rowdy. He had built a homemade potato launcher and had spent one day after school launching potatoes into their subdivision while his parents were gone. The neighbors called the police, and charges had been filed. Although this was the first time that the law was involved, Frank had been breaking family rules for quite some time.

In the initial sessions with the family, the therapist focused on joining with each family member and hearing everyone's side. The therapist acknowledged that Frank's behavior was problematic and observed that everyone—even Frank—wanted things at home to be different. The therapist gradually and respectfully took the focus off of Frank and, through asking about how each person interacted with each other in the family, placed the responsibility for change on the entire family, not just Frank. This provided visible relief to Frank. The rest of the family gradually agreed that everyone could change, and by the end of the second session the whole family was on board.

The family dynamics that contributed to Frank's behavior became clearer as time went on. Roger's attempts to rein-in Frank's behavior seemed actually to be *perpetuating* Frank's behavior. As soon as Roger would come home from work, he would start monitoring Frank excessively, waiting for him to slip up. Roger would correct Frank harshly over the least infraction. Maggie, on the other hand, was constantly trying to smooth over the strained relationship between Frank and Roger. As a result, she was fairly passive in her parenting. She did not have the heart to discipline Frank since he was treated so harshly by Roger, so she let him get away with a lot when Roger was not around. This led to frequent arguing between Roger and Maggie over parenting styles. Ed and Melissa tried their best to fly under the radar and stay out of trouble, but these efforts came at a price. Melissa had started flirting with self-mutilation. Ed was a straight-A student but was very shy and had difficulty making friends. The therapist formed several hypotheses: (1) if Roger would ease up on Frank and start to nurture a positive relationship, Frank would stop acting out in order to rebel against his dad; (2) if Maggie became more assertive, Frank would no longer be able to use "well, Mom let me" as an excuse for his misbehavior. If Roger and Maggie made these changes, the therapist hypothesized that the following changes would occur: (1) the emotional climate of the house would soften considerably, and Ed and Melissa would feel safe to share their concerns with the family— in short, to be kids again; (2) Frank would be more accountable for his behavior and would stop acting out as much; and (3) the entire family would be free to start enjoying each other again, and family unity would increase.

Given the power imbalance inherent in families (i.e., parents have more power than children), the therapist focused on first having the parents change so that their children felt safe to change. Therapy consisted of working toward these goals in couple sessions, and on strengthening relationships in family therapy sessions.

In a couple therapy session early in therapy, Roger was adamantly opposed to the idea that he had anything to do with Frank's acting out. He was convinced that, if Frank just shaped up, the problem would be solved; he was looking for better ways to control his son. The therapist took this as a sign that Roger was in the precontemplation stage, and as a result took a more passive, subtle approach aimed at helping Roger consider that he needed to change. The therapist went with the resistance, giving Roger several behavioral management techniques to try at home. These typically failed, primarily because of the lack of a positive father–son relationship (i.e., Frank did not care about Roger's punishments, presumably because he did not care much about Roger). The therapist validated Roger's frustration and, in an attempt to help Roger look at his role in the problem, gradually started asking Roger to describe *his* relationship with *his* father. As it turned out, Roger's father had been verbally abusive, and Roger had spent most of his time in fear of his father. A partial transcript from a session with Roger and Maggie follows:

THERAPIST: How did it feel to be your father's child?

ROGER: Not very good. I always wondered why he didn't like me. It was like nothing I did was ever good enough.

THERAPIST: It sounds like all you wanted was for your father to be proud of you, but you never got that. It seems like there's still a lot of sadness about that for you.

ROGER: Yeah, there is.

THERAPIST: (*gently*) Roger, if I were to ask Frank to describe his relationship with *his* father—you—do you think he'd say similar things as you said about your father?

ROGER: (*silent for a long time, looking at the floor; after letting out a big sigh*) Yeah, I imagine that he probably would. I'd never thought of it like that. My dad was always so cold; it's hard to think of myself like that as well.

THERAPIST: Well, you've got something your dad never had: a chance to put things right. You could give your son something that you never had from your father.

ROGER: (*quietly crying*) Yeah, I guess you're right.

The therapist correctly recognized Roger as being in the precontemplative stage and used interventions such as dramatic relief to foster insight into his role in the family problems. The next several couple sessions focused on helping Roger foster insight into his efforts to control Frank. As it turned out, Roger was scared to death that he would fail as a father and viewed Frank's truancy as evidence of that. The harder he tried to control Frank—and soothe his own feelings of inadequacy—the more Frank acted out and the worse Roger felt about himself. Roger really caught onto the notion of himself as a person who could break generations of dysfunctional interactional patterns in his family line by giving his children a different experience with their father than he had had with his father. Such self-reevaluation led him into the preparation and action stages.

Roger began trying to connect with Frank. Roger would tell Frank stories of when Roger was a child, and he started taking Frank on his biweekly fishing trips. It was slow going, though, as Frank was wary of Roger's seeming change of heart. Roger frequently got frustrated with Frank's unwillingness to reciprocate Roger's efforts to connect, and Roger vacillated between the contemplation, preparation, and action stages for quite a while. Over time, however, family therapy sessions helped convince Frank of Roger's sincerity and realize his role in his dad's frustration. Frank started to soften toward Roger, which made it easier for Roger to connect. Therapy focused on fostering positive communication, clarifying long-held misconceptions about each other, learning to trust each other's intentions, collaborating on family rules (as opposed to the previous autocratic creation and enforcement of rules), and brainstorming family activities.

As Roger and Frank had more experiences in which Roger would have previously been controlling and Frank would have acted out—yet they did not—their trust with each other began to grow. These changes opened space for changes in other family members as well. Family sessions also focused on helping Maggie became more firm and direct. As she did so, her children started to respect her more, and she gained more confidence in her parenting abilities. Ed and Melissa also felt free to be children now that they did not have to tiptoe around in order to not rock the boat. The therapist worked individually with Ed and Melissa for several sessions to help identify what they were feeling and express that to their parents in family sessions. As they did so, Ed gradually came out of his shell at school and Melissa eventually abandoned cutting herself.

Several variables contributed to the Adamsons' success in therapy, including the fact that the therapist motivated the clients by matching his behavior with each family member's level of resistance. The therapist in this example paid close attention to the stages of change that each family member was in, and successfully used interventions tailored for each stage. Consistent with motivational interviewing, the therapist "led by following," so to speak—by rolling with resistance, being empathetic, and by fostering the desire on the part of family members to move on their own rather than having their alternatives forced upon them by the therapist. Although functional family therapy was not specifically used in this case, its principles of motivation through fostering the alliance with each family member and replacing blame with a relational focus were used to accomplish the same effects that the therapy recommends.

7

A Strong Therapeutic Alliance

The therapeutic alliance underlies all change occurring in psychotherapy and impacts on treatment in numerous ways. At the beginning of psychotherapy, it is *the* key ingredient for most clients in successful (or unsuccessful) engagement, setting the stage for intervention. It also is the vehicle through which almost all treatment strategies in psychotherapy are delivered, whether those interventions are behavioral, cognitive, affect-focused, structural, psychoanalytic, or strategic. Further, it also serves as the central ingredient in determining the acceptability of those interventions by the clients receiving them (Lebow, 1982) and whether between-session homework related to those interventions is carried out (Kazantzis & L'Abate, 2007). The alliance even has a crucial role in affecting decisions about ending therapy; with a strong alliance, clients are far less likely to end therapy until it is completed (Horvath, 2006). Furthermore, in some therapies, such as person-centered, experiential, and psychoanalytic therapies, the alliance itself serves as a major focus of treatment in the process of clients reaching their goals.

To understand how crucial the alliance is in psychotherapy, consider what therapy would be like without a therapeutic alliance. Clients would learn about what might be possible by reading books or watching tapes. The human dimension of treatment would be lost. Although psychoeducation through reading and reviewing materials can and does offer useful information to clients, the human connection is a crucial foundation for success in psychotherapy. In couple and family therapy, the alliance assumes even greater importance due to the multiple participants and accompanying struggles to build several simultaneous alliances and to keep the level of alliance in balance across clients (Friedlander, Escudero, & Heatherington, 2006a).

Much of the impact of psychotherapy, regardless of the therapist's orientation, depends on a client and therapist sharing an alliance as the foundation of treatment. In one research example, Johnson and Talitman (1997), in a study of emotionally focused couple therapy, found that 22% of posttreatment satisfaction and 29% at follow-up was attributable to the couple's alliance with the therapist. A similar impact is also evident even in the most mechanistic of therapies, such as cognitive-behavioral therapy (Krupnick et al., 1994).

In the domain of family therapy, in a fascinating study, Green and Herget (1991) found that the therapeutic alliance and therapist warmth had a substantial impact on outcome even in a strategic therapy centered on consultation with a team, an approach that in its theoretical framework places no importance on the alliance and even actively works to minimize its importance in treatment (Watzlawick et al., 1974). And in another study of strategic family therapy, Stolk and Perlesz (1990) found students in a strategic therapy program to become less effective in their second year than in their first, a finding most parsimoniously explained by the student therapists coming to master the techniques within strategic therapy for *deemphasizing* the therapeutic alliance within their second year. Even the impact of medication is affected. In one of the most influential research studies, the National Institute of Mental Health's collaborative treatment of depression study, the effect of psychopharmacology (studied as a comparison to the psychotherapies included) was greatly affected by the quality of the bond between therapist and client (Elkin, 1994). The human impact of the alliance makes a difference even when the theoretical framework in which the treatment is offered suggests it should not.

Understanding the Therapeutic Alliance

The alliance refers to the quality and strength of the collaborative relationship between client and therapist in therapy (Horvath & Bedi, 2002). There are several essential understandings about the alliance:

• *It is collaborative.* The alliance can be misunderstood as a quality that the therapist brings to the client. However, the alliance is fully interactional and systemic, an operation between one or more clients and the therapist. The most skillful therapist still may not form an alliance with certain clients, either because these clients do not easily form such alliances or because of some gap between the specific therapist and clients. In our experience, we have seen experienced skillful therapists fail to connect with particular clients, only to find those same clients forming a strong alliance with a much less experienced trainee who knows much less about how to intervene but who is a better fit with the clients.

The Smith family formed a positive alliance with their therapist Alice. This might be conceived as simply about the fine job Alice did in bringing warmth, empathy, caring, respect, collaboration, and useful ideas about what to do to the Smiths. However, on more careful examination, their successful alliance formation is better viewed as a dance in which everyone participated. Celia, the mother in the family, brought her own warmth and optimism. José, the father in the family, brought a diligence about being sure everyone made it to each session. And Margarita, the daughter whose acting out caused them to enter therapy, brought along with her challenging attitude a willingness to attend and engage fully in the experience. The alliance co-evolved between the clients and the therapist.

• *And yet, alliances are greatly affected by therapist skill.* Both our observation and considerable research suggest that therapists vary in their abilities to form and maintain therapeutic alliances (Friedlander, Escudero, & Heatherington, 2006c; Greenberg & Pinsof, 1986). We are mindful of one of our colleagues who engages almost all clients and for whom alliances are almost always rated positively (as well of an unfortunate trainee who has had a series of one-session therapies followed by the clients deciding they no longer "need" family therapy). Therapist qualities such as warmth, congruence, and genuineness, described in Chapter 2, and more broadly that which today is called "social intelligence" (Peterson & Seligman, 2004) clearly do on the whole make a difference. So does the therapist's ability to communicate that he or she has seen this problem before, has a plan for how to deal with it, and has had success in the past in helping clients with this difficulty. In one study of family therapy, 45% of the outcome variance was found to be attributable to therapist relationship skills such as warmth and humor (Barton & Alexander, 1977).

Susan has an outstanding record of engaging clients and being successful in working with them. We notice she brings patience, respect for clients, and vitality to her work as well as a keen social intelligence in assessing how to help clients become comfortable in the therapy process.

Probably most therapists with Susan's gift for alliance formation enter the mental health professions with a considerable social skill for intimate personal encounter. We find that therapists who personally have these skills much more readily learn how to build strong alliances. Nonetheless, we also have seen many therapists who personally were less socially skillful who nonetheless learned how to build strong alliances with clients. Sometimes this has been the product of the therapist's own psychotherapy and personal development, sometimes of hard work in the therapy room and supervision developing these skills. We also should highlight that being gregarious and a social butterfly is not synonymous with this ability to establish strong alliances. Therapy is a very special social interaction, depending highly on listening skills, the ability to communicate, patience, optimism, the ability to confront, and the ability to maintain appropriate boundaries. Indeed, we've seen many alliances fail precisely because the therapist was unable to find a comfortable professional role, acting as a sympathetic "friend" more than a therapist.

- *Adapting methods of engagement to the specific client is crucial.* Clients are not all alike. Part of the skill of the successful therapist lies in adapting the methods of engagement and treatment to one's specific clients (Beutler et al., 2005; Lebow, 1987). Some clients expect to hear more from therapists and some less. Some prefer great warmth, others some reserve. Some look to be tracked down when they cancel appointments, while others prefer to be accepted as too busy. Much of the art of therapy lies in understanding and dealing with such differences. For example, Beutler's research (Beutler et al., 2005) suggests that therapist directiveness ideally is tailored to accommodate client reactivity to that directiveness. The message is to be directive to the extent that clients respond well to the therapist's being directive; assume a less directive stance when clients are resistant to influence.

As an aside, this represents the place where therapy manual-based treatments targeted to specific disorders largely fail. Although there are some ways of targeting alliance formation to the presenting problem (for example, engaging in psychoeducation about alcohol and drugs with clients with substance use disorders or communicating the likelihood of difficulty in having the energy to take the first steps in the treatment of depression), the central factors in alliance typically are not about the presenting problem but other aspects of human relating. And clients with different personalities and different family structures respond differently to the range of ways therapists join with them. Alliance formation is more a matter of applying principles of social intelligence as needed than following a preprogrammed set of behaviors.

As an example, Susan is well known in the community of therapists for her warm empathic style. Yet, when she began work with Tom and Mary, both engineers with a limited range of emotion, her warmth quickly came to be regarded by them as an obstacle to engagement. After a single session, they decided to terminate their work with her, asking for a referral. Susan referred them to George, a cognitive-behavioral therapist who brought little emotion to the sessions. Tom and Mary engaged much more successfully with George, with whom they felt more comfortable and went on to work with successfully at their marital problem. Susan remains a fine therapist but was a poor fit with Tom and Mary, who were looking for less of what to most people would be a good quality.

In their work, therapists must always remain well aware of who their clients truly are in order to establish alliance. There is a fine balance between remaining genuine, congruent, and true to oneself in the ways that Carl Rogers described and adapting oneself to the clients in front of you. Working with this balance is one of the major dialectics in the process of therapy. The therapist must remain true to self and yet adapt to the clients seen.

• *Client culture must be considered a crucial aspect of the alliance.* All clients live in a cultural context (Breunlin & Mac Kune-Karrer, 2002). How the therapeutic alliance is best created and nurtured is closely connected to that client culture. The amount of eye contact that is experienced as optimal may be quite different from one culture to another, as is also the amount of physical touching and appropriate distance. Sometimes, simply matching up client and therapist ethnicity may make a difference, especially when clients' socioeconomic circumstances are far removed from the therapist's. This too may vary with clients and therapists. Psychotherapy research suggests that, overall, there is little impact on client outcomes from matching up therapists racially or ethnically to clients (Beutler et al., 2005; Haaga, McCrady, & Lebow, 2006; Horvath, 2001). However, research also shows that learning to speak to issues of a particular cultural group with understanding in language that is accessible minimizes problems attributable to differences. For example, Liddle and colleagues treatment project of inner-city youths with multidimensional family therapy found that emphasizing a boys-into-men theme had a strong positive effect on treatment alliance (Annunziata, Hogue, Faw, & Liddle, 2006).

Amanda had what she thought was a fine first meeting with the Kim family, who had immigrated to the United States 5 years earlier from Korea. She followed her typical protocol for a first session, asking about the presenting problem, being sure to ask questions of all members of the family, and concluding with a prescription for homework based on what she heard during the interview. She was therefore very dismayed when the family called the intake worker after the first meeting to request another therapist. When asked by the intake worker the reason for her request, Mrs. Kim said the principal reason was that Amanda had asked too many questions in too pushy a way and had suggested that life should be "more than just hard work." Amanda had inadvertently violated some of the core beliefs of the Kims' identification with Korean culture, showing little deference to the parents and questioning the family's core values as they related to the benefits of hard work.

One solution for such problems as the one that emerged for Amanda is to be fully conversant with cultural differences. Life experience helps here, but there are also sources of information that can be consulted (Boyd-Franklin, 2003; Falicov, 2003; McGoldrick, Giordano, & Pearce, 1996). Of course, being oversensitive to cultural proclivities can easily result in responding to a stereotype rather than to the family in the room. For example, the Kims as a family could well have fully adapted to and embraced middle-class American ways; it was not possible to know whether this was the case without meeting with them. It is clearly best for therapists to learn about diverse cultures (and find out more about the specific culture if the family has roots in a culture the therapist is unfamiliar with), but to be sure to listen closely and learn from the family about their culture. The simple questions "How was the meeting for you?" and "What might be helpful?" would help avoid misunderstandings like the one Amanda had with the Kims (assuming the therapist recognizes that the answers to these questions also need to be filtered through an understanding of the client's culture).

• *The person of the therapist is a fundamental part of the alliance.* The role of the person of the therapist also must be stressed in the creation of the alliance. Therapists differ as people not just in what they do but also in who they are. Clients react to therapists as therapists but also as people. A therapist has an age, a gender, a culture, a way of speaking and being. These factors all may affect alliance formation.

Chrissie, a 15-year-old who presented with an eating disorder, was assigned to Harvey, a fine 63-year-old clinician. Although Harvey is warm and caring, that he was 63 and a male simply made it impossible for Chrissie to discuss her issues, many of which revolved around sexuality. Harvey had an open discussion about the alliance with Chrissie and offered her the alternative of seeing a student he supervised who was a 26-year-old woman. Chrissie jumped at the possibility and quickly established a great working alliance with Mandy, who, despite having 30 years less experience than Harvey, was in a much better position to work with her. Under his supervision, Mandy successfully carried out the plan for treatment that Harvey created, a plan Harvey could not have carried out by himself.

Here the simple fact is that you can't change such factors as age, gender, and personality. The best course is to match up these factors as best one can in situations where this is likely to matter. In particular, teenagers tend to be very sensitive about gender and often engage better with those closer to their own age. Older adults, similarly, do better in engaging with therapists who have lived for a while. When a treatment involves a mismatch, this is best dealt with in the same way that we described earlier in dealing with culture. Keeping the conversation open about differences, learning from one another, and monitoring the alliance to be sure it is strong enough to support the treatment can enable strong therapies to develop even in these situations. We should also be sure to add that differences do not *necessarily* make for poor alliances. Here we are only describing probabilities. Also, we should emphasize that some experiences in common once thought essential to good alliances and outcomes have been proven by research to really not matter. For example, it once was thought that to treat an addiction successfully a therapist needed to have experienced and recovered from that addiction. Research on alliances and outcomes in the treatment of substance use disorders shows no evidence for this well-known idea (Haaga et al., 2006); whether the therapist has ever experienced recovery firsthand has no bearing on outcomes.

• *Alliances can be subdivided into goals, tasks, and bonds.* The alliance consists of three interrelated parts identified long ago by Ed Bordin (Horvath, 1994; Horvath & Greenberg, 1989; Orlinsky & Ronnestad, 2000). The first part is about the goals of treatment, the ends sought. The relevant questions here are about the extent to which clients and therapists share the same sense of the outcomes that are sought and their expectations about what can be achieved. The second component focuses on tasks, on what is being done in the treatment. The relevant questions here are about the extent to which clients and therapists find what is being done in the treatment appropriate and potentially helpful. The third component of alliance is bonds, the affective connection between clients and therapists. The relevant questions here are about the extent to which clients and therapists feel connected and engaged with one another.

There has been much debate as to how clearly these aspects of the alliance can be differentiated since there always are close correlations among various components of the alliance (Friedlander, Escudero, & Heatherington, 2006b; Horvath, 2006; Knobloch-Fedders, Pinsof, & Mann, 2004). Nonetheless, it remains the case that for many clients the alliances vary across goals, tasks, and bonds (Friedlander et al., 2006; Horvath, 2001; Horvath & Greenberg, 1994). For example, clients may like the therapist and feel attached and agree with the therapist about treatment goals but may nonetheless feel uncomfortable (and out of the alliance) about the tasks employed in treatment.

Stephanie thought that therapy was proceeding well with the Rodriguez family, consisting of mother, father, and three teenage daughters. She felt quite sure of the strength of her alliance because after each session each member of the family thanked her and the mother told her how nice she was. However, after gathering alliance data from the family, utilizing the Integrative Psychotherapy Alliance Scales (see below; Pinsof & Catherall, 1986), she discovered that, while all members of the family felt a strong bond with her, each rated his or her agreement with her about the goals and tasks of treatment poorly. This led to a discussion with the family in which they brought to the surface for the first time their disappointment in the ways that treatment was being carried out. The family felt that too much time was being spent on issues relating to the mother's family of origin and not enough on solving their present problems. This information led to a change in focus by Stephanie to more direct problem solving about how to live better together, and with these alterations the task and goal ratings of the alliance increased over the next few weeks.

The key point here is that the alliance, which can superficially be thought of as just the clients' general feeling toward the therapy and therapist, actually has a number of different aspects. Clients feel a degree of personal connection to the therapist (bonds), a connection about what is being done (tasks), and a connection about where therapy is going (goals). Therapists must remember that, while it may be true that all cylinders are firing in the same direction, it also may be true that the connection is strong in one aspect and weak in another. Obtaining a thorough understanding of each aspect of the alliance enables better practice.

• *Early treatment alliance is highly predictive of how therapy will unfold.* It is hard to overstate the power of early treatment alliance to predict later behavior in treatment. This is especially the case when the alliance early in therapy is not positive (that is, neutral or rated negatively). Ken Howard in several studies with large diverse samples of clients found that if the alliance early in treatment is poor the chances for positive outcomes in treatment become quite small (Leon, Kopta, Howard, & Lutz, 1999). Similarly, in a study of couple therapy early treatment alliance was found to account for as much as 22% of the variance in outcomes (Knobloch-Fedders, Pinsof, & Mann, 2007). Poor early treatment alliance has also been found to be highly predictive of dropping out of treatment (Horvath, 2006). This is not to suggest that a poor early treatment alliance inevitably means a treatment will self-destruct or be ineffective. We believe therapies that begin poorly can recover, but this is likely to happen only if the aberrant issues in the alliance are assessed and addressed.

Tim clearly understood from the complaints of his clients, their coming late to sessions, and their nonverbal behavior that there was a problem in the treatment alliance. This led to an open conversation with the family about the therapy, addressing what they liked and didn't like and their reactions to Tim. Tina, the mother, told Tim that his talking so much during the sessions and his constantly interrupting them was a major problem; the rest of the family agreed. Tim altered his style to allow more uninterrupted conversation within the family, the alliance improved, and the family ultimately succeeded in dealing with their problems.

The take-home message here is that when problems occur early in the alliance they need to be dealt with decisively. A treatment low in alliance needs to be regarded as a treatment likely to end or be ineffective unless some change is made to eliminate the source of the alliance problem.

• *Alliances vary over time. Sometimes the sequence of "tear and repair" can have a strong positive effect on the treatment.* The therapeutic alliance is typically quite stable over the course of most treatment. Once a positive alliance is successfully established, it can readily serve as a vehicle to enable change over long-term therapies or even multiple episodes of therapy (Lebow, 1995). However, the strength of the alliance may vary over time in many treatments. One factor is who the clients are. There clearly are groups of clients that form alliances with more difficulty and for whom the alliance unfolds more slowly, such as clients with borderline personality disorder. There also are client–therapist pairings in which differences in surface characteristics such as race may cause the alliance to take longer to form.

Another phenomenon frequently encountered and documented in both the clinical and research literature is the profound effect of moments in treatment when an event causes the alliance to unravel, followed by repair in which the alliance is restored (Norcross, 2002b). Such events often become powerful positive change events occurring in therapy (Pinsof, 2005). These are not moments that lend themselves to therapists trying to make them occur (the risks of failing to repair the breach are too great), but such moments may make for special opportunities for growth.

As an example, Andre and Therese participated in a couple therapy in which their alliance with the therapist was always rated at the highest level for several months, but they grew no closer to each other. The treatment appeared to be engaging in useful activities, such as communication training and exploration of their genograms, but made no progress. Then, in one session, Steve, the therapist, pushed to explore Andre's passive behavior both in and out of session in a way that led to Andre's feeling challenged and becoming uncomfortable and angry at the therapist. This produced a substantial reduction in his level of alliance, as recorded on alliance scales; Andre even refused to come to the next session. However, after the therapist reached out to Andre and the rupture was repaired through the therapist's apologizing for his insensitivity and through further exploration of the meaning of this event for Andre, not only was the alliance restored but Andre became more available to really work at the issues he brought to therapy, including his passivity. In a sense, it led to his being more engaged in the treatment at a deeper level. The couple's success in working on their problems then moved ahead at an accelerated pace.

Having a positive therapeutic alliance is not a panacea. It sets a helpful tone for treatment and typically leads to success. Nonetheless, sometimes ruptures in the alliance can lead to powerful change events. Of course, they can also lead to the ending of treatment or less subsequent work. These are moments of challenge that can lead either to gains or the dissipation of energy in treatment.

• *Alliances in couple and family therapy vary across family members in a complex way.* As we noted in Chapter 3, in couple and family therapy multiple alliances must be considered. Each client has his or her own separate alliance with the therapist. This complication, itself, makes for other complexities because in couple and family therapy not only the strength but also the balance among the various alliances matters. In particular, when there is a split alliance in which the alliance with one partner (in couple therapy) or family member (in family therapy) is strong and the other partner or another family member is weak, the chances for poor treatment outcomes may rise exponentially (see below).

As we described earlier (in Chapter 3) Pinsof (1995; Pinsof & Catherall, 1986) has emphasized the importance of attending to aspects of alliance building in couple and family therapy beyond the multiple individual alliances involved. In his categorization of couple and family therapy alliances, Pinsof suggests that the alliance within the therapy system as a whole often differs from the clients' individual alliances with the therapist. For example, a couple might each as individuals feel a bond with the therapist and a positive alliance but might not feel such a set of links with the therapist as a couple together.

Pinsof and colleagues (Knobloch-Fedders et al., 2004) also point to the need in couple and family therapy to consider the alliances within the couple or family itself (apart from the therapist) as part of the understanding of the alliance in couple or family therapy. It is hard for therapy to succeed with a low level of alliance among family members as a unit with one another in a treatment. This represents a major problem in much couple therapy, where some alliance between the couple to work on problems is clearly a necessary condition for change in most cases and where that alliance is likely to be tenuous early in therapy. The same problem emerges as well in family therapy, such as when there is no alliance within the parental coalition in the presence of an acting-out adolescent. And even in individual therapy, Pinsof, Zinbarg, and Knobloch-Fedders (2008) have shown that the individual's perception of there being a felt alliance between the others in her or his life (who had no contact with the therapist) and the therapy had a strong positive effect in predicting continuation in therapy.

Men's alliances with the therapist may be particularly important in couple and family therapy. The effects of differences in alliance between men and women can be complex. Knobloch-Fedders et al. (2007) found in research assessing couple therapy that when men's mid-treatment alliances were higher than their partner's, positive outcomes were more likely; and outcomes were more closely related to women's ratings of their partner's alliance than to their own level of alliance with the therapist. It may be that (given the frequent finding of greater engagement by women in all forms of therapy) indications that the male in a heterosexual couple is successfully engaged may be the strongest predictor of favorable outcomes in couple therapy.

Establishing and Maintaining an Alliance in Couple or Family Therapy

How, then, does the therapist best establish and maintain a therapeutic alliance? This represents a question that no manual describing psychotherapy can speak to well because the alliance is the result of collaboration between the client and the therapist. What works to establish an alliance with one set of clients will differ substantially from what will work with another.

For example, picture two families who are in treatment in order to obtain help with an adolescent's substance abuse problem, a frequent target of empirically supported therapies that include family therapy. One family, the Markovs, values direct communication and speaking about difficulties. Another, the Jankowskis, has a history of never speaking about problems, and its members feel a great deal of discomfort in even referring to its difficulties, let alone investigating what lies behind them. The best process for establishing alliances with these two families would vary considerably. In the first, an open stance by the therapist and leadership in engaging in open discussion would likely help to establish an alliance, but in the second family such an approach early on would likely lead to an early termination due to the discomfort that ensued. Alliance building involves "different strokes for different folks." A therapist's skills in understanding and empathizing with individual family members trumps any specific behavioral steps for establishing a therapeutic alliance with families.

Nevertheless, one may list a number of specific therapist behaviors that enhance alliance formation. Although such behaviors are often recommended as part of specific approaches to evidence-based practice, this set of skills transcends any particular model in which they are named. There clearly are a generic set of behaviors in couple and family therapy that typically help build the alliance (with, of course, the caveat already presented that it is the meaning of those behaviors in each particular family that matters and that meaning may be idiosyncratic in any given family).

Tracking the Alliance

At the top of this list of therapist behaviors that help form the alliance is attention to the alliance itself. That is, some tracking of the alliance formally or informally early in treatment makes a considerable difference. As we have noted, Howard and his colleagues showed in their progress research conducted in large samples receiving individual psychotherapy that if an alliance was not successfully formed by the fifth session, it was unlikely treatment would be successful (Greenberg & Pinsof, 1986; Howard et al., 1991; Kolden & Howard, 1992). The therapist can simply ask about the alliance and observe client behavior or employ an instrument that assesses the alliance, such as Pinsof's couple and family therapy integrative psychotherapy alliance scales (Knobloch-Fedders et al., 2004) or one of Duncan and Miller's simple alliance measures consisting of only one to four items (Miller, Duncan, Sorrell, & Brown, 2005).

Pinsof's self-report integrative psychotherapy alliance scales assess alliances along two dimensions. The first dimension is goals, tasks, and bonds, as described earlier. The second dimension includes the alliance between the client and the therapist (called self-therapist), the felt sense of the quality of the alliance between the others in the family and the therapist (called other-therapist), the quality of the alliance as being experienced between the whole system and the therapist (called group-therapist), and the alliance experienced between the members of the family system themselves (called within-system). There are individual, couple, and family versions of the scales now included as part of the Systemic Therapy Inventory of Change (Knobloch-Fedders et al., 2004). The scales, in their second major version, have proven highly reliable and valid as measures of alliance. These most recent versions of the integrative psychotherapy alliances scales are included in Appendix B.

The Miller–Duncan Session Rating Scales for measuring alliance are far simpler, with four items asking for an assessment of the alliance on a line continuum (Miller, Duncan, & Hubble, 2005). This brevity of the scale makes it more subject to problems in reliability than longer scales (item response can vary radically from session to session, based on random error) but has the advantages of both simplicity and expeditiousness in the clinical process and thus is very easy to integrate seamlessly into treatment. The most recent versions of the Session Rating Scales for adults, children, and young children are presented in Appendix B. Working copies are free for personal use and available for downloading at *www.talkingcure.com*.

Such instruments provide the therapist access to simple quantitative data that readily assess with almost all clients whether the alliance is going well or poorly and with whom. Both Pinsof and Duncan and Miller employ their instruments in the clinical context as an intervention in treatment. Clients and therapists collaboratively view the clients' alliance scores and in so doing are spurred to discuss the alliance, both how it is working and how it might be improved.[1]

In general, the expectation is that the therapeutic alliance will be strongly positive in psychotherapy. Even "middle-of-the-scale" ratings as satisfactory for client–therapist alliances are the exception among those who continue treatment beyond the first few sessions (Lebow, 1982). In part, this predisposition stems from the intrinsic nature of a positive alliance in such an intimate activity as psychotherapy and, in part, from those with low levels of alliance terminating early in treatment. This pattern also is typical in couple and family therapy (Friedlander et al., 2006). Here, the tendency toward an overwhelmingly positive response is slightly lessened by the presence in these therapies of individuals who do not themselves seek out treatment and continue because of the strong alliance of another family member with the treatment (Friedlander et al., 2006; Horvath, 2006; Horvath & Bedi, 2002; Norcross, 2002b).

When exceptions appear where the alliance is poor, either assessed through information provided in session or through alliance questionnaires, special attention to the problems in the alliance is required. When alliances do emerge as lower than would typically be expected, the therapist should assess whether this is the product of specific problems in the case that would be likely with any variation

---

[1]Friedlander and Heatherington also offer an excellent system for rater rating of couple and family therapeutic alliances: the System for Observing Family Therapy Alliances (SOFTA; Friedlander et al., 2006b; Friedlander, Escudero, Horvath, et al., 2006). These instruments have excellent reliability and validity, but because they require the taping of sessions and raters these instruments are better suited to research than clinical work.

in the therapy or whether some change in the therapy might be likely to work better.

In such a context, there are many useful questions to ask oneself and/or the clients. Is there some other way of approaching the clients? What are the constraints to a better alliance? Are goals, tasks, or bonds, principally involved? Is the problem pervasive across all clients or confined to one client or one subsystem? Does the alliance appear to be more a matter of the nonspecific factors involved in the treatment, or is it failing because the intervention strategy is a poor fit with the clients or not working (again, remembering that common factors are interrelated with the specific treatment involved)?

Because no change is likely without a strong therapeutic alliance with all clients, the situations in which the alliance should be allowed to remain at a low level are few and far between, mostly reserved for those instances where the therapist must convey an unpopular essential therapeutic message (e.g., "You must face that you have been violent in your marriage"). Even in these instances, some minimal level of positive alliance remains a requisite for successful treatment. Moments that involve "tear and repair" can be highly impactful, but such an impact is far less likely if a positive alliance did not precede these moments. In mandated treatments, where the alliance with the referral source such as the court may have transcendent importance in guaranteeing that the treatment will continue, there may be more leeway for periods of low levels of alliance, but even in such instances change remains unlikely without a positive alliance (Lebow, 2005). Methods such as motivational interviewing have been developed in part to allow for some substantial chance to build a therapeutic alliance when clients begin with low levels of motivation and/or cannot see the problems that require attention (Miller & Rollnick, 2003). In general, such methods are aimed at building alliance rather than confrontation early in treatment (Haaga et al., 2006).

Joining Behaviors

Minuchin (1974) and numerous others after him have described a broad range of therapist behaviors that help alliance formation in couple and family therapy. The reader is especially referred to Minuchin and Fishman's (1981) encyclopedic description of specific behaviors that help overcome barriers to forming alliances with families.

Joining can involve as simple a process as utilizing both language and behavior that respect and are perceived as comforting within the client system and culture. For example, the use of expletives may be a source of joining in one family and yet represent a constraint to joining in another. Similarly, whether speaking to the family from a position of authority or as a coequal collaborator may affect the formation of an alliance with the family, depending on the nature of the particular family.

Specific efforts to enhance other common factors in treatment such as instilling hope also add to alliance formation. Most clients are demoralized about their problems at the beginning of treatment, and to the extent the therapist can help create a reality-based optimism about the change process, alliances grow. This is a point where the common factors we discuss in this book build on one another to create a global positive gestalt about treatment, ultimately impacting on both the mediating and the longer-term goals of treatment.

The technique of reframing (Robbins, Alexander, Newell, & Turner, 1996; Sexton & Griffin, 1997), which aims to envision problems in a new, less pathological and blaming light (and one of the most frequently encountered techniques in couple and family therapy), specifically often proves very helpful in moving from being dispirited to a more positive view of the therapy. More broadly, the same is true of creating a solution-oriented focus that aims at accomplishing the same mediating goals (O'Hanlon & Beadle, 1997). For most clients, speaking of solutions and the likelihood of reaching them helps to create a positive alliance. Yet, so can any approach that brings a new, more hopeful viewpoint to the problem's resolution. The same effect can be enabled by a mutual focus on family of origin, emotion, a behavioral plan, or inner experience. The key skill here lies in knowing which strategies are likely to be the most acceptable ones that mutually satisfy the clients' needs—and when to change strategies if initial efforts fail (Lebow, 2006a; Pinsof, 2005). A wide array of therapist behaviors, ranging from providing support to self-disclosure, can encourage alliance building. The skill lies in making certain that the behavior remains genuine and is appropriate to the family in treatment. Here, as elsewhere in this volume, we underscore that it is ultimately the common factors rather than the specific approach that matters most, even though advocates for specific approaches might point to the unique and special qualities of their methods.

The Split Alliance

Of special importance in couple and family therapy is the split alliance. Couple or family therapy frequently begins with one party more invested in the therapy process than the other(s), or at least with one party lesser motivated to engage. There may be a couple in which one partner wants to improve the marriage and the other has little interest, or a family in which the parents strongly wish to see change in the behavior of an adolescent, whereas the adolescent simply wants to keep doing what he or she is already doing. In such instances, a split alliance often develops in which family members differ considerably in their alliance with the therapist. A split alliance can also develop over the course of therapy when family members come to experience different levels of joining by the therapist.

Split alliances are very challenging even for the most skillful of therapists. On the one hand, there is the need to keep the alliance with the allied clients(s). Typically they are the ones that are causing the treatment to continue, and radical shifts to engage the other party might well lose the therapy altogether if such shifts lead to a loss of alliance with those clients. Yet, the work of the therapy is unlikely to proceed well without engaging the less engaged clients. So, the task becomes to look for ways that respect the ongoing process of the treatment and the alliance with the allied parties and yet can reach out to and involve the less engaged clients. Family therapists have for many years pointed to the parallel needs to maintain a strong alliance with the person who brought the couple or family to therapy and to the simultaneous need to ensure that alliances are balanced by paying special attention to building the alliance with the less involved family member (Minuchin, 1974; Whitaker & Keith, 1982).

Efforts to change position and side with the less engaged clients for the sake of alliance are not likely to prove helpful. The therapist does best to maintain an ethical position in treatment and side with one family member's version of what may be helpful over another only when the therapist's ethical compass points in that direction. Ultimately, as Rogers (1961) suggests, alliance depends on therapist genuineness and congruence (see Chapter 2). More useful are efforts to redirect attention to ways of experiencing that join better with the less allied clients or that utilize language or a manner of discussion that does so. In this way, alliance can be built without impinging on the positive alliance already present or presenting what the therapist actually believes to be a distorted message to the family (it's also crucial to remember that there are occasions that what the therapist thinks to be a short-term plan to join with someone is followed by termination and, thus, the therapist's final word on the subject, an experience likely to be repeated often).

As elsewhere, direct discussion of the alliance problem also typically is helpful. A curious nonjudgmental attitude on the part of the therapist is useful. For example, he or she might review each client's alliance scales over the past few meetings and be curious about what has been experienced and what might be done about it. Clients are often the best source of information for what they need to form strong alliances.

The Zadins presented for therapy due to Tom, age 17, being arrested for marijuana possession. Over the first few sessions, it became clear both through examining alliance scales and in session process that whereas Jan, the mother, was highly engaged in treatment, Ron, the father, and Tom were not. In the next session the therapist opened a discussion about how useful the family was finding the treatment. Ron and Tom both reported there was little of the kind of discussion they found useful, suggesting that the sessions were too full of "feeling" language. While not abandoning the family's basic need to face feelings (which in part was why the meetings were engaging for Jan), the therapist moved to more "guy-centered" discussion of practical ways to fix problems. She also began each session with a short conversation about the success or failure of the local baseball team, which Ron and Tom both followed closely. The alliance issue was soon resolved, and the family became able to truly work collaboratively on the problems that faced them.

Assertive Engagement

One extremely useful finding from the research on alliance in family therapy is the value of assertive engagement with families who do not typically undertake mental health treatments. Assertive engagement represents active efforts to go out and build alliances with clients, in contrast to the passive intake call, first session, and subsequent response to clients' frequently showing their ambivalence about treatment by dropping out early from therapy. In assertive engagement, therapists develop an active strategy for engaging the family; often, with families who do not naturally seek out therapy, home visits to establish alliances are involved.

The therapist explores who is most available to build an alliance and who might be most powerful in being able to bring clients to therapy. Building an early treatment alliance with that person or persons is crucial. The answer to this question is likely to lie with a parent in a family presenting with difficulty such as conduct disorder in a child or adolescent. However, in the population of Cuban American families in which Szapocznik and colleagues developed these procedures of assertive engagement (Mitrani, Prado, Feaster, Robinson-Batista, & Szapocznik, 2003; Santisteban & Szapocznik, 1994; Santisteban et al., 1996; Szapocznik et al., 1988), the therapists first strategized primarily about ways to engage the acting-out adolescents into treatment since they held particularly powerful positions in these families. Szapocznik's research confirmed that following such methods of assertive engagement increased engagement from about 20% with ordinary passive intake procedures to 75% in these families. The take-home message here is that in couple and family therapy typical traditional intake procedures often must be supplemented or replaced by a more active engaging procedure.

Intervention as a Method of Building Alliance

Common factors and specific treatment factors are often represented as entirely separate and distinct. This makes for an exciting horse race in which the proponents of specific methods and common factors argue for who really has the data to support their argument. Although we believe the data do in fact overwhelmingly demonstrate that common factors contribute a great deal more to treatment outcome than specific treatments (Norcross, 2002b), we suggest that a moderate common factors viewpoint makes the most sense—precisely because these common and specific factors systemically influence one another, just as systems theory describes (Bateson, 1972; Boszormenyi-Nagy & Spark, 1973; Bowen, 1974; Straus, 1973). Good intervention that makes sense to families feels helpful and engages and therefore leads to better therapeutic alliances, just as such alliances lead to better outcomes. Typically, there are many specific paths by which such intervention can prove effective, but it is important to be on one of them. To the extent that intervention is not engaging or experienced as helpful, alliance suffers and early termination becomes likely. And to deliver any treatment in sufficient doses to have any lasting effect, a strong therapeutic alliance is necessary. No treatment can be effective if clients do not attend to and engage with the treatment closely over an extended period of time.

The Significance of the Therapeutic Alliance

The therapeutic alliance has a special place in the practice of psychotherapy. Of all the aspects of treatment that have been subject to research in relation to treatment outcomes, it has the most and best evidence for support. Although the concept of the therapeutic alliance was somewhat late in entering the discourse about couple and family therapy, alliances in this context are clearly just as important as in the world of individual therapy.

However, alliances in couple and family therapy are far more complex than in individual therapy. The therapist must remain focused on not only the multiple individual alliances of the clients with the therapist but also with the relative strength of those alliances, with their alliance as a group working together with the therapist, and even with their alliances with one another in treatment. The building and maintenance of therapeutic alliances over the entire course of the therapy must always be in the spotlight. Therefore, asking about alliances, observing less direct signs of alliance or its erosion, and/or actively using instruments to measure the strength of alliances are all essential ingredients in successful couple and family therapy. When the therapeutic alliance is strong, the power of active therapeutic ingredients in treatment is greatly enhanced. When it is weak, treatment rarely lasts long enough to deliver the strategies for change thought most essential by the therapist, much less for those strategies to be accepted by the clients and experienced as helpful.

8

Models

All Roads Lead to Rome

There are almost as many models of relational therapy as there are therapists. Is each of these models truly unique? If they are different, do those differences matter? If they are similar, is there any clinical relevance to the similarities? One of the main tenets of our common factors approach is that different models use different language to talk about the same distressed and healthy relational processes, and use linguistically different but pragmatically similar interventions to help move a system from distress to health. In other words, when working with a couple or family, most relational models start at similar conceptual places, often walk down linguistically different but pragmatically similar intervention paths, and arrive at the same place. An emotionally focused therapist working with primary emotions (Johnson, 2004) and an integrative behavioral couple therapist eliciting soft emotions (Jacobson, Christensen, Prince, Cordova, & Eldridge, 2000) both constitute examples of this.

On the other hand, we do believe that some models emphasize different aspects of relational processes (e.g., emotionally focused therapy emphasizes affect while narrative therapy emphasizes cognitions) or use interventions unique to that model, yet have the same net result on the couple or family. In other words, despite starting at the same point sometimes models take different (yet sometimes intersecting) paths that lead to the same destination. This is in keeping with the systemic concept of *equifinality*—the tendency for similar results to be achieved within a system from different initial conditions and in many different ways. Systems theory applies even to the system of systemic therapies!

Another main tenet of our common factors approach is that it is better for a therapist to be thoroughly familiar with several different couple and family therapy models as opposed to just one so that the therapist can adapt to the client rather than vice versa (Blow et al., 2007). We believe that the trick to mastering diverse couple and family therapies, then, becomes seeing through the model-specific language to the common starting lines (i.e., conceptualizations of distress), common pathways taken (i.e., interventions), and the common finish lines (i.e., conceptualizations of health). Once a therapist can do this, he or she is not bound to one particular model and the couples or families that will respond well to that model. Rather, he or she is free to pick and choose from several different models to find the approach that fits the client the best, and yet still maintain a focus on the same relational processes.

Thus we come to the purpose of this chapter, which is to illustrate how different models conceptualize the same systemic processes underlying health and dysfunction and recommend similar interventions to help a couple or family move from dysfunction to health. We add this chapter to other excellent works that aspire to the same goal, most notably Dattilio and Bevilacqua (2000) and Dattilio (1998). We begin with an illustrative vignette, followed by a discussion of what we described in Chapter 3 as a factor common to all systemic models, namely, interactional cycles (Davis & Piercy, 2007b). Using interactional cycles as the systemic backdrop, we provide model-specific explanations of common processes that create and maintain distressed interactional cycles. Using the same relational models, we then discuss diverse model-specific interventions that share the goal of altering affective, behavioral, and cognitive aspects of interactional cycles. We end with a discussion of common aspects of a healthy couple's interactional cycles.

We do not attempt to provide an exhaustive list of healthy and distressed relational processes and common interventions, nor do we discuss every model of couple and family therapy. Rather, we hope to present a new way of thinking about couple and family therapy models with the hope that the ideas presented here can serve as a springboard for future practice, training, research, and writing on this issue.

Luis and Alida, a middle-class Hispanic couple in their 30s, presented for therapy with "difficulties communicating." When Sara, their therapist, asked them to elaborate, Alida described her frustration over trying to get Luis to "help with the new baby and come to bed at a decent hour so he isn't so tired and grumpy all day." Luis and

Alida had just had a new baby, and Alida, a homemaker, was feeling overwhelmed with caring for the baby and their other young child. She looked forward to Luis coming home each evening so he could help her, but lately Luis had been coming home later and later, and when he did come home he did not want to spend much time with the family. Instead, he would eat dinner, help a little with the dishes, and then disappear into the garage or his office until as late as 5 o'clock in the morning. Alida often woke up at night and, realizing he was not in bed, would feel hurt and lonely and cry herself back to sleep. She was beginning to lose trust in him, as he was often vague about what he was doing at night when she could not find him. She also felt resentful that he got to spend so much time doing "whatever he wanted" while she spent all day attending to the needs of their two small children. She felt increasingly abandoned and tried to get Luis to be more involved by making more and more demands of him. Whenever she talked to him, it was to try to get him to do something differently.

When Sara asked Luis to explain why they were coming in, Luis said that he was under a lot of stress at work. He was self-employed, and his landscaping company had been struggling due to a recent downturn in the housing market. His employees and customers were getting increasingly anxious, and he said that he spent all of his day "trying to get people to not be mad at me." He saw himself as letting people down "in every aspect of my life," and the more stressed he felt, the more he wanted to avoid everything. Since home was so stressful, he did not want to come home to more stress. When he did come home, he could barely wait for everyone to go to bed so he could "have some peace and quiet and finally not worry about having to make other people happy." Inevitably, however, the more days that Luis stayed up late, the more tired, unproductive, and irritable he became. He was feeling increasingly helpless and out of control.

As Luis and Alida described their interactions around this issue and others, it became apparent to Sara that their behavior fell into a typical pursue–withdraw pattern in which Alida pursues and Luis withdraws. As Alida grew increasingly frustrated with what she saw as Luis's "irresponsibility and lack of concern for my feelings," she would respond by trying to convince him to come home earlier. That was not working. In exasperation, she had recently accused him of "being a selfish jerk" and "a failure as a husband and father." Frustrated with her seeming inability to get Luis to understand her plight, she said, with tears in her eyes, that she had recently threatened to move out unless Luis "could get himself together."

Luis, on the other hand, viewed Alida's disappointment as a reminder of one more area in his life in which he was failing. The more she "complained and nagged," the more frustrated and inadequate he felt, and the more he withdrew in an attempt to "figure out how to solve the problem" or to simply avoid the relationship altogether. On the rare occasions when he did speak to Alida, it was usually an angry outburst "to get her to stop nagging." Both Alida and Luis felt alienated and unloved, thought their partner did not care about their relationship, and behaved in ways that exacerbated the very stance in their partner that they were frustrated about.

Sound familiar? While the words of the song may change, the music behind Luis and Alida's dance is played every day in countless therapists' offices across the world. There are almost as many models for helping Luis and Alida out of their predicament as there are therapists to implement those models. We will apply a few of these models to Luis and Alida through our common factors lens.

Common Distressed Relational Processes and Treatment Goals: Interactional Cycles and Patterns

Though there are obvious exceptions to this rule (e.g., physical violence, organic disorders, etc.), a staple of all systemic approaches is the notion that each person's response to any given situation within the system is understandable given the responses of the others in the system. Interactional cycles form as the affective experience, behavioral responses, and cognitions of one partner both influence and are influenced by those of the partner. For example, Luis and Alida's interactional cycle formed a pursue–withdraw pattern, with related affect, behavior, and cognition as illustrated in Figure 8.1. Alida's pursuing becomes understandable when viewing Luis's withdrawing, and vice versa. Whereas a linear view of their relationship would label Alida as an overdemanding wife and Luis as an uncaring husband, a systemic approach claims that each partner is trying to make the relationship work the best they know how and that their attempted solutions to the relationship problem are actually the problem. To induce change, every systemic model focuses on altering the affect, behavior, and/or cognitions of at least one participant in an interactional cycle with the assumption that doing so will induce similar change in the other person in the interactional cycle.

An interactional cycle between two people offers at least six points of possible intervention: each partner's interpretation of the other partner's actions, intentions, and so forth; each partner's behavior; and the emotions experienced by each partner (see Figure 8.1). For example, Luis thinks that he will never be able to satisfy Alida (cognition), feels inadequate (affect), and avoids home as a result (behavior). In response, Alida thinks that Luis does not care (cognition), feels abandoned and rejected (affect), and criticizes Luis as a result (behavior). Each of these six elements perpetuates the others. Similarly, changes in any of these six elements that Alida and Luis view as related to their problem will likely trigger changes in the others—which, if orchestrated correctly, will likely result in the cycle beginning to shift from destructive to healing. For example, if Luis sees and experiences Alida as scared and lonely, he will likely treat her more kindly than if he thinks she is a nag. She may in turn be more supportive of him in his stressful situation, which may increase the chance that he will be more supportive of her, and so forth. Therefore, in an effort to shift the interactional cycle from being destructive to healing, systemic treatments share one or more of the following

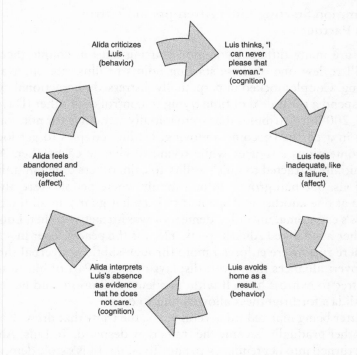

FIGURE 8.1. Luis and Alida's distressed interactional cycle.

goals (Sprenkle & Blow, 2004a): (1) to help each partner interpret the other's actions differently (i.e., a change in cognition); (2) to help each partner behave in a way that ameliorates rather than exacerbates the problem (i.e., a change in behavior); and (3) to help each person feel differently about him- or herself and his or her partner (i.e., a change in affect). See Figure 8.2 for an example of a healthy interactional cycle.

From interactional cycles, however, systemic models seem to part ways, each rushing to linguistically different parts of the systemic conceptual frontier and each staking a claim on its seemingly unique patch of land. Little wonder that there is resistance to our common factors approach, then, since we claim that they all end up living in the same place! There is just not that much new systemic territory to be discovered.

Model-Specific Conceptualizations
of Common Distressed Relationship Processes

A Common Starting Line: Attempts to Control One's Partner

There are many different common starting lines in couple therapy; we will review one of these starting points to illustrate our way of thinking. Couples locked in perpetually distressed interactional cycles often spend a great deal of time trying to control each other (Davis & Piercy, 2007b). Attributes that were initially attractive (or not noticed at all) in a partner become annoying, leading couples to get locked into contentious struggles while trying to change each other. Alida was initially attracted to Luis's ability to calm others down in difficult situations. She had grown up in a family where people were always yelling at one another and she had to keep her guard up all the time, so Luis's easygoing, unruffled demeanor was attractive to her. Luis, on the other hand, liked Alida's spunk. He was the peacekeeper in a family where rules were enforced more through subtle nonverbal threats and covert alliances than overt displays of anger. Part of him wanted to be free to express himself without silent retribution, and he found that Alida's forthrightness allowed him to do so.

After being married for several years, the traits that drew them to each other gradually became the traits they despised. To Luis, Alida's spunk turned into her tendency to nag. To Alida, Luis's stoic demeanor morphed into his tendency to withdraw from difficult conversations.

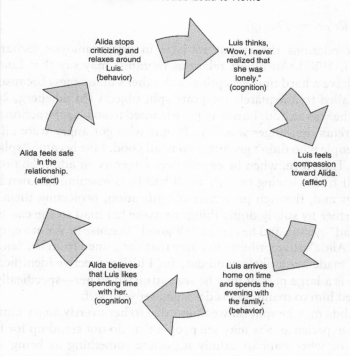

FIGURE 8.2. Luis and Alida's healthy interactional cycle.

As their mutual efforts to try to control each other brought about more of the attributes they despised, they gradually began to believe that resigning themselves to a miserable relationship was the only option if they were to stay married.

Linguistically Different Paths: Model-Specific Conceptualizations

Though most models share the goal of helping partners become less controlling and more accepting of differences, the conceptualization of *why* the tendency to control exists (or if answering "why" even matters) varies widely. Understanding the theoretical explanation of the existence of the cycle is important, as it provides a coherent rationale for the interventions to follow. We have deliberately selected three couple therapy models that are quite different philosophically in order to illustrate common interventions among diverse models.

Object Relations Therapy

Object relations theory has its base in psychoanalysis (Scharff & Scharff, 1987). An object relations therapist may say that Luis and Alida have a hard time accepting each other's uniqueness because they have failed to adequately integrate split objects (Middleberg, 2001). When he was a child, Luis may have learned from his interactions with his parents that anger was bad. People who got angry were all bad, and people who didn't get angry were all good. Luis became "split" on anger. Therefore, when he experiences anger as an adult, he protects himself from viewing himself as all bad by disowning his own angry feelings and, through projective identification, projecting them onto his partner by subtly doing things to make her mad so she can be the "all-bad" person and he can be "all-good" because he is not angry and she is. Alida's susceptibility to anger that she gained from her family of origin made her a likely candidate for Luis's projective identification, which is a large part of why he was attracted to her—specifically, she allowed him to maintain his damaged sense of self.

Alida may be split on weakness due to her overtly angry family of origin experience. She may see people that do not stand up for themselves or who want to calmly negotiate something as being weak. Since the "weak" part of herself was continually shamed in her family of origin, she has not owned her own weakness and thus recruits Luis to hold it for her in a similar pattern, as described above for Luis.

Therefore, object relations theory would say that Luis and Alida are intolerant of each other's differences because of their own poorly developed internal representations of self and other. To accept the other's differences they would first have to own their disowned aspects of the self that their partner is carrying. It is not *their partner's* anger or weakness that they do not like—it is *their own* anger or weakness that they do not like. In other words, they will continually require that their partner carry the disowned aspects of their self until they learn that anger and weakness—and therefore an angry or weak person—is neither all good nor all bad. Until each partner takes responsibility for his or her own anger and weakness, he or she will continually try to change his or her partner.

Emotionally Focused Therapy

Emotionally focused therapy has its base in attachment theory (Bowlby, 1988). An emotionally focused therapist may say that Luis and Alida are insecurely attached, which makes it difficult for either to trust that the partner will foster a secure base in which he or she can safely express his or her emotional needs. A person's attachment style (generally referred to here as secure or insecure, although there are many types of insecure attachment) develops from one's early interactions with caregivers. From birth through adulthood, a person is continually asking the question "To what extent can I count on others to be available and responsive when needed?" A securely attached person learns early in life that he or she can generally depend upon others to meet his or her emotional needs and consequently that his or her needs are legitimate. Conversely, an insecurely attached person learns early in life that others cannot be depended upon to meet his or her emotional needs. Through repeated dismissal or rejection of those needs, he or she comes to believe that those needs are invalid and that expressing them to others carries a high risk of painful rejection.

People interpret events in a way that confirms their attachment style. Therefore, an insecurely attached person may view differences in his or her partner as evidence that the partner will not adequately love him or her, and subsequently he or she will try to get rid of those differences through controlling behaviors. Despite this, most people want to connect with significant attachment figures such as their spouse. If the partner is insecurely attached, however, an interactional cycle will form in which that person simultaneously seeks and fears closeness. An emotionally focused therapist believes that emotions are the strongest signal of these attachment needs, and a person simultaneously seeking and fearing a safe emotional experience will display harsh, distancing secondary emotions such as anger the more that he or she feels softer primary emotions such as sadness and fear. Sadly, however, the display of secondary emotions sets in motion an interactional cycle in which the partner responds in turn, thus ensuring that the emotional closeness that he or she desires is never obtained (Johnson, 2004).

Solution-Focused Therapy

Unlike object relations and emotionally focused therapists, a solution-focused therapist would not be concerned about historical events that may explain the role that attempts to control play in Luis and Alida's distressed interactional cycle (deShazer, 1988). In other words, "why" does not matter! The client is the expert on his or her life—not the therapist. Even if the therapist and couple agreed on a "why," first of all there is no way to know that that is *really* the reason, and second of all, so what! The problem is still there, and it needs to be dealt with in the present moment. That is best done by enlisting Luis and Alida's underutilized strengths by helping them to recognize times in the past when he or she has dealt with this problem successfully, and encouraging him or her to replicate what he or she did at the time. The "problem," then, is that Luis and Alida are not seeing their own strengths and utilizing their own resources to get out of their mess. A solution-focused therapist would view lengthy historical explanations of what is wrong as an unhelpful diversion that actually further disempowers the couple by amplifying their shortcomings.

Linguistically Different but Pragmatically Similar Paths: Model-Specific Interventions

In addition to understanding the "why" (or whether the "why" even matters) behind attempts to control one's partner, it is also important to understand the "how," or the interventions used to help a client progress from distress to health. Though the interventions that flow from the theory-specific conceptualizations sound different, and in some cases *are* different, they share the same goal of helping each partner be less controlling and more accepting of his or her partner's differences. Furthermore, these interventions frequently overlap in their efforts to alter the interactional cycle by changing behavior, altering cognitions, and getting clients to experience emotions differently.

Some models will focus on one aspect of the interactional cycle more than others (e.g., emotionally focused therapy will focus more on the emotional aspect while solution-focused therapy may focus more on the cognitive and behavioral aspects). Whichever aspect of the cycle the model orients the therapist to does not seem to matter so much as the fact that it focuses on the cycle in some systematic way that is meaningful to the clients and the therapist (Davis & Piercy, 2007b). Furthermore, the distinctions among various shifts in cognition, affect, and behavior are likely to be at least partially artificial. For example, if an emotionally focused therapy client hears one's partner expressing him- or herself from a position of vulnerability and responds in turn, can it be said that cognitions and behaviors did not change as well as emotions? The same could be said for an object relations client who comes to interpret the motive behind his or her partner's actions differently and as a result feels differently toward him or her and starts treating him or her more kindly. Whether changes in affect, behavior, or cognition come first makes a lively theoretical debate, but it is likely a matter of theoretical nuance that disappears when tailoring an approach to client preferences.

Similar Interventions: Changing Behavior

A solution-focused therapist may help Alida and Luis behave in a less controlling way through interventions such as *solution-oriented discussion*—an overall atmosphere focused on solutions rather than problems (Furman & Ahola, 1994). Questions that contribute to this atmosphere as Luis and Alida are encouraged to change their behavior by focusing on their strengths include "If you were to do something different the next time the problem presents itself, what would you do?" (Furman & Ahola, 1994, pp. 54–55). Other interventions such as the *formula first session task* (deShazer, 1985) also help clients explore healthier behavior. In this intervention, Luis and Alida would be encouraged to watch for things in the family between the first and second sessions that they'd like to continue to have happen. For example, Luis may notice a time that he comes home on time, and Alida may notice a time that she is kind where she normally would have been angry. They would be encouraged to repeat those situations.

In object relations theory, Luis and Alida must gain insight into their problems before lasting change can take place. Therefore, most of the interventions are aimed at increasing cognitive insight around their controlling behaviors (discussed later). Once that insight is gained, however, Luis and Alida would be encouraged to translate that new insight into new behavioral patterns of relating to each other (Scharff & Bagnini, 2002). Luis might be encouraged to express his anger through assertive rather than passive-aggressive communication, while Alida might be encouraged to reach out for help more when she is feeling inadequate or incompetent.

Since emotionally focused therapy is an experiential model, having Luis and Alida interact differently is a critical component of treatment. In fact, the core emotionally focused therapy intervention is *restructuring interactions*. This is often done using an *enactment*, in which the therapist will have one partner say to the other something like "Can you tell him, 'I'm afraid that when you come home late, it means you don't want to be with me. So, I'm going to shut you out. I'm not going to let you devastate me again'" or "This is the first time you've ever mentioned feeling inadequate. Could you tell her about that inadequacy?" (adapted from Johnson & Denton, 2002, p. 35). Enactments are thought to introduce a new way of experiencing internal emotions as well as cementing new behavioral interactional patterns. In the context of an enactment, Luis may be encouraged to show Alida his feelings of inadequacy rather than stonewalling, while Alida may be encouraged to show Luis her fear of abandonment. The assumption driving both interventions is that doing so would invite a "softer" response from the other, thus setting in motion a healing interactional cycle.

Whatever the intervention used, the assumption of most systemic models is that if people *behave* differently around each other, the way they *think about* each other and *feel toward* each other will also shift.

Similar Interventions: Altering Cognitions

A solution-focused therapist uses many interventions to help Alida and Luis alter cognitive aspects of their interactional cycles. With the *exception question* (deShazer, 1988), Luis and Alida are encouraged to search for times in the past when the problem was not a problem. Are there times when Luis came home on time or otherwise showed that he cared? Are there times when Alida has approached Luis in a way that helped Luis want to be around her? In addition to the behavioral effects mentioned above, the exception question helps clients shift from thinking that their partner is *always* a certain way, potentially opening up cognitive space for a softer view of their partner. A solution-focused therapist may also address cognitions when using *scaling questions*. Luis and Alida, for example, would be asked to identify a number between 1 and 10 that represented their current situation. If they picked 3 and the higher numbers would indicate where they wanted to be, the therapist would then ask, "What would you be thinking differently if you were a 5?" Luis and Alida would then be encouraged to think the things they would think if they were a "5." The same routine could be repeated for matters relating to behavior and affect.

An object relations therapist relies heavily on cognitive interventions by *offering insights into possible unconscious conflicts* that are contributing to the interactional cycle. For example, an object relations therapist might say to Alida, "You learned to disown your vulnerable parts because showing hurt in your family of origin brought you shame and humiliation" (Middleberg, 2001, p. 350). Or the therapist might say to Luis, "I wonder if it is easier to have Alida hold your anger than it is for you to own it, because it would be too painful to think of yourself as being an angry person." These new insights are aimed at helping Luis and Alida view their role in the cycle differently, thus helping them understand that it is each of *them* that needs to change rather than the partner. Helping Luis and Alida gain insight into their unconscious motivations frees them from blaming each other for their problems and opens the path to an unencumbered exploration of new behaviors.

An emotionally focused therapist also uses several different interventions to restructure a couple's cognitions. *Empathic conjecture* or *interpretation* is similar in form to interpretation in object relations therapy. In these interventions, the emotionally focused therapist may say things like "You don't think it's possible that anyone could see this part of you and still accept you. Is that right? So, you have no choice but to hide?" (Johnson & Denton, 2002, p. 235). The purpose of this intervention is to "clarify and formulate new meanings, especially regarding interactional positions and definitions of self" (p. 235). In other words, its purpose is to alter cognitions in the hope of altering the interactional cycle.

The assumption behind all of these cognitive interventions is that if Luis and Alida can *perceive* each other differently, their *actions toward* and *feelings about* each other will also change, thus setting in motion a healing interactional cycle.

Similar Interventions: Experiencing Emotions Differently

The role of emotions in solution-focused therapy has been a source of debate, with some saying that traditional solution-focused therapy is too cognitive and sterile (Kiser, Piercy, & Lipchik, 1993; Piercy, Lipchik, & Kiser, 2000), while others disagree (Miller & deShazer, 2000). Regardless of which side is right, there is nothing inherent in solution-focused therapy that prevents emotional processing. Kiser and colleagues (1993) suggest that solution-focused emotional processing can be done by *joining with negative emotions* in order to shift the focus to positive emotions. For example, a therapist could say to Luis and Alida, "Things certainly seem to be going from bad to worse. Do you think they have hit rock bottom yet? What do you imagine things will be like at their worst?" (Lipchik, 1988, p. 136). Clients will often say that things are not as bad as they could be yet, which gives the solution-focused therapist something positive to work with. Kiser et al. (1993) also note that the *miracle question* (deShazer, 1988) can be altered to focus on emotions in addition to behaviors and/or cognitions. In the miracle question, Luis and Alida are asked to imagine life after an overnight miracle has occurred that wipes away their problems. To focus on feelings, this question could read: "Suppose that one night, while you were asleep, there was a miracle and this problem was solved. How would you know? Would you feel different? How could you let your husband/wife know that you were feeling this way?" (Kiser et al., 1993, p. 236). This question may open up space for a different emotional experience between Luis and Alida.

The role of emotions is central to object relations therapy, particularly in regard to *transference* and *countertransference*. Transference refers to Luis and Alida's shared feelings about the therapist. The couple's transference elicits countertransference—emotions, behaviors, and ideas from the therapist. The therapist's countertransference is then used as a source of data about Luis and Alida's unconscious, with particular weight given to a therapist's emotional countertransference, since "the emotions roused in [the therapist] are often nearer to the heart of the matter than his [or her] reasoning" (Heimann, 1950, p. 82). This emotional countertransference becomes a major source for offering insights to the clients—one of the main object relations interventions. For example, the therapist may say to Luis, "When you feel inadequate in your ability to care for your family, it reminds me of how you felt as a boy when your father would criticize you for trying to build something on your own" (adapted from Middleberg, 2001). Luis would then be free to realize that it was his dad he had issues with rather than Alida, and he could then choose what to do with those issues.

Not surprisingly, an emotionally focused therapist focuses primarily on emotions! The majority of emotionally focused interventions are directed toward helping Luis and Alida access, identify, and express their primary (rather than secondary) emotions to their partner, which tends to elicit the same from their partner, thus instigating a healing shift in their interactional cycle. *Evocative responding* helps clients expand previously unexplored aspects of their emotional experience. An emotionally focused therapist might say: "Alida, I noticed that when you talked about Luis coming to bed late, your voice dropped a bit and you dropped your head. What was going on for you at that moment?" (adapted from Johnson & Denton, 2002). *Reframing* emotional processes in the context of the interactional cycle and attachment processes serves a similar purpose. The emotionally focused therapist may say, "Luis, you're afraid that you're letting her down, and you can't stand to feel her disappointment that confirms that, so you stay away, right?" This can help Alida see the "softer" motivations behind Luis's withdrawing, thus helping it feel safer for Alida to be vulnerable with Luis.

Regardless of the model-specific interventions used, most systemic models focus on helping couples identify, understand, and reprocess emotions in the hope that healthier interactional cycles will result. In Luis and Alida's case, the intent is to help them stop trying to change—through pursuing and withdrawing—the aspects of their partner that they don't like.

A Common Finish Line: Appreciating One's Partner's Differences

As we mentioned earlier, most relational models help clients end up at similar places. We provide one possible common finish line here. In this example, most relational models share the belief that as a partner abandons attempts to control his or her partner and instead embraces and enjoys his or her partner's differences, negative interactional cycles will shift and the relationship will begin to flourish. Some researchers have suggested that the ability to see a partner's quirks as endearing virtues to enjoy rather than annoying habits to extinguish is a chief hallmark of a mature marriage (Markman, Stanley, & Blumberg, 1996). Gottman and Silver (1999) similarly notes that all marriages have unsolvable problems—issues that are going to be around for as long as the marriage exists—and that successful marriages are those in which partners learn productive ways to communicate about those problems rather than continually expecting their partner to change in a way that will presumably make the problem go away.

Again, different models speak about this change in different ways. An emotionally focused therapist (Johnson, 2004) might say that the couple has fostered a more secure attachment and therefore no longer perceives the partner's differences as a threat to their mutual security in the relationship. An object relations therapist (Scharff & Scharff, 1987) might say that the couple has integrated split objects into a more complete self and therefore does not perceive the partner's difference as a threat to his or her self. A solution-focused therapist (deShazer, 1988) would not have a complex explanation for what happened—only that the couple has been empowered to reach its goals by rediscovering ignored strengths. A cognitive-behavioral therapist (Dattilio & Epstein, 2003) might say that the partners have a more adaptive schema of relationships and that as a result interactions around problematic issues are now more rewarding than punishing. A narrative therapist (White & Epston, 1990) might say they have adopted a more open and less restrictive story about themselves and each partner. A Bowenian therapist (Kerr & Bowen, 1988) might say that the increased tolerance of difference reflects higher differentiation. The list could go on and on. The point is, most systemic models strive to have couples and families shift the emotional climate from one that controls and restricts its members to one that nurtures autonomy.

Additional Common Processes of Distressed and Healthy Relationships

Using the systemic concept of interactional cycles as a backdrop, we have provided one example of how diverse models conceptualize common processes of distressed couples, utilize overlapping and distinct interventions to ameliorate those processes by focusing on affect, behavior, and cognition, and lead a couple toward similar ends. We believe that the same line of thinking can be applied to any distressed relational process. Fortunately, there is a large body of research on the commonalities of distressed and healthy couples (Gottman & Notarious, 2000). Most marital and family therapy models address these common processes, even though they use different language to describe them. For example, the ability to hear a partner's point of view without becoming defensive or emotionally flooded has been shown to be predictive of marital satisfaction (Gottman, 1994). A Bowen therapist (Kerr & Bowen, 1988) may describe the difficulty in doing this as low differentiation; a cognitive-behavioral marital therapist (Dattilio & Epstein, 2003) may note automatic thoughts that trigger defensiveness and say the couple needs to challenge these and learn self-soothing techniques; an internal family systems therapist (Breunlin, Schwartz, & Mac Kune-Karrer, 1997) may say that the clients need to learn how to have their wounded, reactive parts step back when triggered by their partner's wounded parts and let their self lead. Whatever they call it, therapists embracing most models believe that similar processes need to change, have similar ideas of what that change will look like, and use mostly overlapping yet some unique interventions to help the couple effectuate that change.

9

A Meta-Model of Change
in Couple Therapy

The Need for a Meta-Model of Change

Common factors research is often critiqued as consisting of nothing more than general concepts (e.g., a good therapeutic alliance is positively related to outcome) and lists of variables that do little to guide therapy and research in a systematic way (Sexton & Ridley, 2004). We believe that those critiques are valid but that they reflect the status of the *current* common factors literature, not the promise of the overall movement once it is developed further (Sprenkle & Blow, 2004b). To date, the main categorization of the many proposed common factors variables has been *broad* and *narrow* (Davis & Piercy, 2007a; see also Chapter 1), with broad variables being those inherent in the process of therapy itself (e.g., the therapeutic relationship) and narrow ones being those aspects of therapy directly tied to the uses of a model (e.g., the shared goals of changing affect, behavior, and cognition). We believe that the lack of a substantial common factors framework explaining how these variables may interact to produce change has led to a number of misguided ideas within the common factors world. For example, it is not uncommon to hear a common factors proponent say "The therapeutic alliance is of supreme importance!," as if the alliance is both necessary *and* sufficient for effective therapy and that other aspects of therapy can be ignored. "Since all models work the same, models don't matter!" is, in our opinion, another misguided notion that is often batted around in common factors circles. We believe that prominent variables such as the therapeutic alliance

123

are vital to successful therapy but that they produce change in concert with several other variables, including the structure provided by a good model. (See Chapter 5 for more mistaken views of common factors.) To say that one variable is more important than the other is, as our colleague Dr. Adrian Blow observes, "like saying the engine is more important than the tire!" Can you really say that a car will work properly that has one but not the other?

On one hand, the lack of a coherent model of common factors is understandable, given that a main point of the movement is that the last thing we need is another model! A common factors model could go against the very principles upon which it is based. On the other hand, we agree with the critiques that broad lists of common factors do not do much to help guide clinical teaching, practice, or research. For example, if all that good therapy consisted of was forming a good relationship or offering a credible ritual to address problems, then why employ therapists at all since religion, for instance, provides both of those things? Independent of one another, individual common factors provide an incomplete picture of change.

So, what is to be done to reconcile the two? We believe it is possible to organize the broad and narrow common factors that have empirical support into a meta-model—a "model of models," so to speak—that can be used to guide change regardless of which model is being utilized. Such a model would not just be another model; it would not simply rewrap the same old stuff in a different package. Instead, a common factors meta-model would ideally provide a framework that could be superimposed on the work of diverse therapists working with diverse models with diverse clientele. Such a model would integrate broad and narrow common factors into a coherent principle-based explanation of therapeutic change that would find applications in a wide variety of clinical circumstances. A meta-model could orient a therapist to issues that he or she could be attending to regardless of which model of therapy he or she was using.

To be useful, such a model would have to be broad enough to allow for the variation, flexibility, creativity, and different maneuverings expected from diverse therapists, clients, and models and yet narrow enough to provide clinical, training, and research guidance. If a model were too broad, it would not help therapists to know what to focus on and when, leaving them lost with only a vague map to guide them. It would be like trying to find your way around New York City with only a map of the major highways in New York State. If the model were too specific, the therapist could get lost in the details or get too caught up in trying to remember what he or she was "supposed" to be doing, which might stifle the therapist's creativity, the unique needs of each client, the client's feedback, and the natural flow of good therapy. It would be like trying to cross the United States with hundreds of maps that detailed every slight gradation of the ground's surface. By focusing on minutia, the map would be a hindrance rather than a guide.

An ideal model would provide enough detail to allow a therapist to know what he or she should be paying attention to and why at any given time across diverse circumstances, and yet be broad enough to allow for conceptual and interventive flexibility with each unique client. The purpose of this chapter is to outline an empirically derived meta-model of common factors of couple therapy that we believe fits that description.

Empirical Development of the Model

The development of this model started as my (S. D. D.)'s doctoral dissertation in Virginia Tech's marriage and family therapy program under the direction of Dr. Fred Piercy. I wanted to find therapists that practiced "pure" model-specific therapy and then see if I could derive what commonalities characterized their practices. I assumed that if there were commonalities detectable among theoretically distinct practices, then those commonalities might be part of the golden thread that runs through effective therapy. I assumed that if I found commonalities there would be similar ones evident among the practices of other therapists as well. I thought that couple therapy model developers would fit the "pure" practice that I was looking for, and model developers Dr. Susan M. Johnson (emotionally focused therapy), Dr. Richard C. Schwartz (internal family systems) therapy, and Dr. Frank M. Dattilio (cognitive-behavioral couple therapy) were kind enough to give me access to them and some of their couple clients that had been successful. I also recruited some of their former students and clients on the assumption that these practices might represent an average clinician's practice more closely than would the developers' practices.

I asked the model developers, their former students, and the successful couple therapy clients of each a series of questions regarding their experience in couple therapy. I then used qualitative analysis techniques to search the interviews for common practice patterns as well as to provide an explanation for how those patterns interact to contribute to successful outcomes. Due to space constraints, we will not use many direct quotes from the study to support each concept, but interested readers can find further elaboration in the work of Davis (2005) and Davis and Piercy (2007a, 2007b).

How Narrow and Broad Common Factors Interact to Produce Change in Couple Therapy: A Meta-Model

The model (see Figure 9.1) is outlined in a sequential order (i.e., from conceptualization to intervention to outcome). This is in part because such a linear explanation is unavoidable when explaining separate phenomena in writing (i.e., one has to come first, second, and third). It is also because that is generally how therapy naturally progresses, and that is how the participants in the study described it. Keep in mind, however, that the progression through each of these stages is more circular—one stage informs and is informed by the other—than linear. For example, the conceptualization phase is interventive in that it gives the clients hope. Also, there is no distinct line between where the intervention phase ends and the outcomes start; they often co-occur. Similarly, the order of the "cognition, affect, and behavior" elements of the intervention stage is arbitrary; we do not claim that one must precede the others for change to occur.

The Beginning Stages of Therapy: Adopting a Model

At least two phenomena characterize the beginning sessions of therapy. First, at some level, clients are confused as to how to help their relationship. Efforts to change on their own have failed. They cannot see a way out of their problem. As Frank and Frank (1991) note, clients coming into therapy are "conscious of having failed to meet their own expectations or those of others, or of being unable to cope with some pressing problem ... [and] feel powerless to change the situation or themselves" (p. 35). Second, through their model of therapy, therapists have a clear idea of what is "dysfunction" in a couple, what is "health," and how he or she can get his or her clients from the former to the latter. They know how to help. Therefore, a main goal of the beginning sessions of therapy is to help clients replace their current chaotic, "stuck" view of their relationship with the hopeful "there is a way out" view that the therapist's model gives them. We will discuss how to do that successfully later.

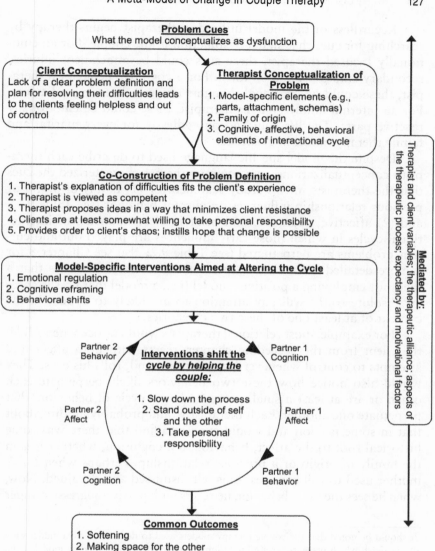

FIGURE 9.1. How model-dependent (i.e., narrow) and model-independent (i.e., broad) variables combine to create change. From Davis and Piercy (2007b). Copyright 2007 by the American Association for Marriage and Family Therapy. Reprinted by permission of Blackwell Publishing.

Regardless of the model utilized, a therapist begins therapy by searching for cues that signal dysfunction in the couple. For an emotionally focused therapist, these cues could be attachment injuries, secondary emotions, and so forth. For a cognitive-behavioral therapist, these could be irrational thoughts and self-defeating behaviors. For an internal family systems therapist, these could be emotionally reactive parts. The list could go on endlessly for every marital and family therapy model in existence.

Despite the model-specific language used to describe each therapist's conceptualizations, two common themes characterized the cues that the therapists in this study searched for (1) family-of-origin or previous relationship influences on current behavior (see Table 9.1); and (2) affective, cognitive, and behavioral components of interactional cycles in which those early influences are played out and current problems are perpetuated (see Table 9.2; also see Chapter 8 for a more detailed discussion of interactional cycles). The cues that a therapist employing a positivist model (i.e., a model that presupposes an absolute truth) will pay attention to are likely to appear in the context of at least one of these two categories.[1]

For example, most relational therapists would notice when Alida, the client from the preceding chapter, reacts with both anger and attempts to control whenever Luis, her husband, rolls his eyes. They would also notice how these two behaviors likely perpetuate each other, or are at least a small part of a larger cycle of behaviors that perpetuate one another. Each therapist would probably inquire about that in some fashion and would expect to find that there was some historical root to the affect, behavior, and cognition, whether it is in the family of origin or a previous relationship. Perhaps when Luis's mother used to roll her eyes, Luis felt dismissed and devalued. Now, when he sees the same behavior, he reacts with passive-aggressive anger

---

[1]It should be noted that the couple therapy models used to derive this meta-model were all positivist, which presents certain limitations. Postmodern couple therapy models (e.g., solution-focused, narrative) will be conceptually different from positivist models (e.g., emotionally focused therapy, cognitive-behavioral therapy, internal family systems therapy). For example, early relationship influences on current relational behavior is a common area of conceptualization in our model. Postmodern models are not concerned with a client's early relationship influences on their current relationships. Future research investigating commonalities of postmodern approaches may shed light on conceptual similarities and differences from positivist models and whether these differences matter. We anticipate that there may be more conceptual differences between postmodern and positivist models, but that those differences would disappear when intervening and both models would lead to similar changes.

TABLE 9.1. Common Conceptualizations: Family-of-Origin Experiences

Verbatim explanation of change	Theory specific explanation of change	Common factors explanation of change
Dr. Johnson (EFT): "I don't think my clients had a very supportive environment to grow up in."	*EFT:* Family-of-origin experiences form a person's attachment style—a set of beliefs about whether or not the "self" is lovable. Different attachment styles have unique characteristic emotional displays that serve the function of maintaining a level of emotional distance the person is comfortable with. Insecurely attached couples simultaneously seek and fear emotional closeness.	Early life experiences shape the way a person acts, thinks, and feels in adult intimate relationships. These feelings, thoughts, and behaviors can serve to establish a close nurturing relationship or to distance and alienate. Dysfunction in one aspect (i.e., affect, behavior, or cognition) will be associated with dysfunctions in the others.
Dr. Dattilio (CBT): "He dealt with ... [his childhood feelings of] being rejected ... and the way his wife acted sometimes reminded him of the way his father acted."	*CBT:* Family-of-origin experiences form a person's scripts and schemas—core beliefs about the world and themselves in relationships. Behavior and emotion in relationships are driven by the cognitions that form their schemas. People will arrange their relationships in a way that reinforces their schemas.	
Ms. O'Neil (IFS): "She had been ... sexually molested by her brother, ... and ... her mother had a fairly significantly abusive part."	*IFS:* Internal "parts" form as a result of early trauma. These parts are always characterized by extreme emotions, behavior, and thoughts. A part's primary function is to protect the "self," though as a person grows older the parts interfere with the establishment of healthy relationships.	

Note. CBT, cognitive-behavioral therapy; EFT, emotionally focused therapy; IFS, internal family systems therapy.

and refuses to come to bed with Alida, instead staying up late into the night. Perhaps when Alida's father would behave passive-aggressively, Alida's mother would turn her head and roll her eyes in disdain and then later talk to Alida about how weak her father was for getting so angry. For both Luis and Alida, their behaviors, cognitions, and affect perpetuated their partner.

TABLE 9.2. Common Conceptualizations: Interactional Cycles

Verbatim explanation of change	Theory specific explanation of change	Common factors explanation of change
Dr. Johnson (EFT): "They would sometimes both attack, but basically their negative cycle is that he would sort of shoot and run and withdraw."	EFT: Becoming emotionally vulnerable enough to establish an intimate relationship is too scary; so, insecurely attached people will maintain emotional distance through harsh secondary emotions. These emotions evoke similar emotions from the partner and serve to emotionally alienate each partner from the other.	Each partner's thoughts, feelings, and behaviors both influence and are influenced by those of their partner's. Distressed couples will form an interactional cycle in which each partner's dysfunctional cognitions, affect, and behaviors are reinforced. If partner's thoughts, feelings, and/ or behaviors are modified, the cycle will shift from destructive to healing. Shifts in one aspect will lead to shifts in the others.
Dr. Dattilio (CBT): "She had to learn to stop giving in to [her husband]. The other end of it was to teach him what to do with his own insecurity and volatility."	CBT: People interact with others in a way that reinforces the beliefs that constitute their core schemas. If these schemas contain irrational beliefs about relationships, interactional cycles will form that perpetuate those beliefs.	
Ms. O'Neil (IFS): "Her part was making her interpret] behaviors in a negative ways, ... which then didn't really allow ... her to have any access to his self or her own self."	IFS: One person's parts— which are inherently emotionally reactive—tend to elicit their partner's parts, which are also emotionally reactive. The goal is to have the client's self—which is inherently calm—guide communication rather than the parts.	

Note. CBT, cognitive-behavioral therapy; EFT, emotionally focused therapy; IFS, internal family systems therapy.

Therapist Credibility

Therapist credibility often first comes into play with the referral source. When a client receives a strong referral for a particular therapist, that client often begins therapy assuming that the therapist will be able to help. These clients begin therapy assuming that it will work, and a therapist's competence bolsters that assumption. But what is "competence"? In this study, therapists were viewed as competent largely because they provided viable explanations of the clients' problems (i.e., through the therapist's model) that the clients believed and—through their nonanxious presence and the fit of their model to the clients' problems—gave the clients hope that the therapist had encountered similar problems before and could provide a reliable way out. Knowing that the therapist is comfortable with the process and has seen "the other side," so to speak, gives clients a reason to take the risks that good therapy requires.

A therapist's passion for his or her model is another important component of therapist credibility and client engagement (Blow et al., 2007). For therapy to be effective, both the therapist and the client have to "buy into" the clinical approach that is offered. The therapist's passion for his or her approach can influence whether clients truly engage with the processes and procedures favored by the model, which—provided these address realistic aspects of the relational distress that the couple is experiencing—will help the clients ultimately achieve their goals.

Fit of the Model with the Couple's Experience

Couple therapy is largely about therapists offering a healthier way of thinking, feeling, or behaving, and the clients integrating that into their existing ways of relating to each other. If, to some, that may come across as too therapist-centric, we think that that is unavoidable. By using his or her model to guide what to focus on, let pass by, reframe, and so forth in the couple–therapist dialogue, a therapist gradually introduces to the couple new ways of looking at their relationship problems. The clients will likely "buy" the therapist's conceptualization if they view what is being said as relevant to their problems and they can sense that the therapist believes what he or she is talking about. The conceptualization will help if it deals with realistic aspects of relational health and dysfunction (e.g., having a couple hang a crystal over their door may help some couples feel lucky, but it isn't likely to do anything for chronic marital conflict!). A relational therapist does not necessarily have to sit down and literally "teach" the model to his or her clients; rather, the model is often taught indirectly through the conversations and interactions between the clients and the therapist.

Establishing a Climate That Minimizes Resistance

Successful marital therapy begins in a climate that minimizes client resistance and fosters a sense of safety. This favorable setting is effectuated through the therapist's monitoring and influencing several key dynamics. Successful therapists strike a balance between the *structure* (i.e., therapist direction and guidance) and the *flow* (i.e., unstructured client processing) of a session. A couple's level of emotional reactivity can be used to determine the structure–flow balance. Highly emotionally reactive couples need more structure in order to provide a safe environment until they learn to regulate their emotions enough to interact with each other in a healthy way. Healthier couples often find too much structure intrusive, making attempts at healthy communication choppy and frustrating (Butler & Bird, 2000; Davis & Butler, 2004).

Establishing a climate of *neutrality* also helps to minimize resistance, regardless of which model is being used. Neutrality refers to viewing *the relationship* as your client rather than either individual within the relationship. With the relationship as the client, therapists will be pushing each person within the relationship to make changes. Focusing unduly on one partner often leaves that partner feeling attacked and the other feeling justified in maintaining his or her part of the problem. Neutrality is monitored and maintained over the full course of treatment as well as on a session-by-session basis. I (S. D. D.) often tell my couple therapy clients during the initial session that their relationship is my client and that there will often be days when one of them feels more in the "hot seat" than the other—but that is for the greater good of the relationship. I also encourage them to let me know if they feel as though I am continually focusing on one of them to the exclusion of the other. I have found that this discussion circumvents a lot of hurt feelings as therapy progresses.

Provided that the clients view the therapist's methods as relevant to their problem, *repetition* of those methods also serves to establish a sense of safety. Repeating techniques and interventions that clients are finding useful helps couples integrate the new skills and thoughts into their lives, thus increasing the hope that they will get better. Of course, this is true regardless of the model being used.

Motivational Beliefs

In Chapter 6 we discussed the notion that all clients are motivated—the therapist's task being simply to match his or her interventions to the clients' level of motivation so that their motivation increases rather than decreases. Therapist credibility, the fit of the model to the couple's experience, and a climate that minimizes resistance by attending to the level of client motivation all seem to add to the couple's hopes that therapy will work. Additionally, motivational beliefs and metaphors help to give clients a context within which to justify the difficult work of therapy. Such beliefs offer a "big picture" that provides direction and purpose to a client's hopes, thus amplifying their motivation. Some of these beliefs are presented by the therapist, often as a reframe of the couple's struggles. Others are beliefs that clients already possess. In the study, some clients mentioned the belief that each setback presented an opportunity to grow even closer to the partner than before. Others mentioned that their therapist said, "This is going to get worse before it gets better" or "You'll have issues that you bring to the table that cause problems—no matter whom you're married to—so why not resolve them now?" Regardless of where the clients' beliefs originated, the important thing was to give them the motivation to resolve their problems in their current relationship, no matter how difficult the work became. Motivational beliefs helped make the work seem worthwhile even though it was challenging.

Client Willingness to Take Personal Responsibility

"I wouldn't yell so much if she'd get off my back!" "I wouldn't have had an affair if he wasn't so cold!" Many clients enter couple therapy attempting to use their partner's bad behavior to justify their own. Although this can be an understandable response, clients must be willing to acknowledge that they share at least some blame for their problems if their relationship is to improve (with some obvious exceptions such as abuse). There are things that a therapist can do to foster even small amounts of this willingness to take responsibility, but for any interventions to work clients must first be willing to acknowledge that they need to change—even if they do not know what or how to change.

Alida and Luis (the couple discussed in Chapter 8) came to therapy confused and hopeless. They had each tried to solve their problems the best they knew how, but the harder they tried to fix things, the worse the situation became. They did not know how or if therapy could help, but because Sara, their therapist, came well recommended, they decided to give it a try. Though the beginning of their first session was awkward, they soon relaxed as Sara listened to and validated each of their experiences. They had also expected Sara to panic when she heard their problems—*they* certainly felt panicked. They were pleasantly surprised, however, when Sara remained calm and yet connected to them. Her unruffled response helped them feel safe—perhaps there was a way out! By the end of the first session, Alida had begun to see Luis as stressed and overwhelmed rather than insensitive and uncaring; Luis had started to see Alida as lonely and frightened rather than cold and nagging. Though they still had a long way to go, the new view of each other that had started to take root gave them hope that perhaps there was a way out of this emotional maze that they had not previously considered. They felt like they were in the right place.

Luis particularly liked that Sara was interested in how he felt; he had worried that he would "get into more trouble" in therapy by simply being told more things to change. Alida liked that Sara validated her feelings of loneliness. Alida had started to wonder whether she was expecting too much and should just settle for what she had. Sara had a wonderful way of letting things get intense enough that Luis and Alida could say what they were really thinking and feeling—but not so intense that they did not feel safe. They also liked that Sara would readily point out things they could do differently; this practice helped them to know that Sara would not deliberately take sides, thus making it a lot easier to accept her feedback.

As the couple begins to adopt the therapist's conceptualization of their problem and to feel hope, they continue working on their challenges regardless of which model the therapist is using. In addition to the common processes during the early stages of therapy, we believe that there are also commonalities to the interventions used by diverse models once therapy gets underway. These commonalities will be the focus of the next section.

The Intervention Stage: Raising Awareness of and Altering Each Person's Role in the Cycle

Relational therapists using diverse models implement various interventions unique to their model but aimed at the same ends. As we discussed in Chapter 8, most interventions are aimed at altering affective, cognitive, and behavioral elements of the interactional cycle between the two partners, although some models emphasize one aspect more than others (see Table 9.3). Either way, most relational therapists intervene by helping clients become aware of their role in the interactional cycle and helping them change the role they play.

For example, an emotionally focused therapist would *primarily* be mindful of how the display of secondary emotion perpetuates the

TABLE 9.3. Common Interventions: Altering the Cycle

Common interventions	Representative quotes	Common factors explanation
Emotional regulation	*Paul (EFT client):* "Before therapy we were able to talk about feelings in a way that we accused each other. Now the difference is ... that ... each of us talks about how we feel in the situation without accusing the other partner."	Once clients were aware of the cycle and their role in it, therapists helped the clients know how to change in order to initiate a healing interactional cycle. Therapists accomplished this by helping clients regulate their emotions, reframe cognitions, and shift behaviors. Though therapists from each model focused on certain aspects more than the others (e.g., EFT practitioners focused on emotion more, and CBT proponents focused on cognition and behavior more), all therapists focused on each of the three aspects in helping their clients exit destructive interactional cycles. Shifts in one aspect almost always co-occurred with shifts in the others and almost always achieved the same end of helping the clients exit the destructive cycle and begin a healing cycle.
Cognitive reframing	*Tiffany (CBT client):* "Therapy taught me to ... step back and say, 'What am I doing here that I can do differently that might make the outcome of this more positive? Maybe he's reacting to me because he was brought up a certain way. Maybe my behavior isn't the best right now and I'm contributing to the escalation of whatever it is that's going on.' ... I'll step back and say, 'Okay, maybe I did something or said something that was really interpreted poorly.'"	
Behavioral shifts	*Bridgette (IFS student):* "Beth told me that when you're washing the dishes and you're worrying about 'what's out there that needs to be done and what about this application and what about this form, what about this messy house,' then is the best time to climb in bed and read a book or take a bath, because then 'I gain perspective and can talk with my husband calmly again.'"	

Note. CBT, cognitive-behavioral therapy; EFT, emotionally focused therapy; IFS, internal family systems therapy.

cycle—Luis's withdrawing invites Sara's contempt, and vice versa. Interventions will be fashioned to help each partner identify, own, and express his or her primary (e.g., hurt and fear) rather than secondary (e.g., anger, contempt) emotions, assuming that the expressed primary emotions will evoke the same from the partner, thus setting in motion a healing interactional cycle that allows the partners to resolve their attachment injuries (Johnson, 2004).

On the other hand, a cognitive-behavioral therapist would *primarily* focus on the automatic thoughts, schemas (i.e., deep-seated cognitions about relationships), and behaviors that perpetuate the cycle (Dattilio, 2005). He or she would help clients explore alternative explanations of and responses to their partner's behavior, which would in turn alter the cycle. An internal family systems therapist (Breunlin et al., 1997) would pay attention *primarily* to cognitive and emotional aspects of the cycle. He or she would help each partner explore the beliefs associated with each "part" that was reacting so strongly to the other partner's "part." This approach would help them explore different ways of interacting with each other.

Although the entry point into the cycle varies, all systemic models focus on altering an aspect of the cycle. Based on the findings of the study, and contrary to conventional model-specific wisdom, we believe that the most effective point of entry into the cycle—be it cognitive, affective, or behavioral—is determined more by client preference than the objective superiority of one point over the other (e.g., emotions versus cognitions). We hypothesize that *a change in one aspect of the cycle will be associated with changes in the others*. Perhaps the most important element of systemic intervention is not *which* aspect of the cycle a therapist focuses on but rather that the therapist focuses on one aspect that fits with the clients and that the therapist intervenes in a systematic way.

Regardless of the therapist's entry point into the cycle, most of his or her interventions serve the following purposes (see Table 9.4): (1) to slow down the process; (2) to help the couples "stand meta" to themselves in the cycle, thus experiencing themselves and their partner differently; and (3) to encourage personal responsibility by changing the partners' stance in the cycle. We will discuss each of these concepts in more detail below.

Slowing Down the Process

Couples often enter therapy locked in contentious struggles to change each other. The first step in altering an interactional cycle is to help couples slow down this process—to help them switch from their typical "autopilot" responses to more productive interactions. This step can be accomplished in several ways, including encouraging the clients to take a deep breath, structuring the amount of time each person

TABLE 9.4. Common Interventions: Raising Awareness of the Cycle and Each Individual's Role in It

Common interventions	Representative quotes	Common factors explanation
Slow down the process	Louise (EFT client): "Over time ... our therapist wouldn't let him go on that long and she would say, 'Look at Louise—what's going on here? Why do you think she is being quiet?' and that sort of thing ... pointing out something he might not have been aware of himself and trying to help him not interrupt." Bridgette (IFS client): "My therapist kept inviting me back to where I was instead of letting me run forward."	Therapists focused on helping each client be aware of his or her role in the cycle and change his or her stance in it. They did this by (1) slowing down the process; (2) helping clients stand meta to themselves and their partner; and (3) encouraging personal responsibility in changing their stance in the cycle. Metaphors were often used to help clients keep a "picture" of the cycle in their minds as they worked on altering the cycle inside and outside of therapy.
Stand outside of themselves and their partner	Geller (CBT client): "We were communicating better and seemed to step outside ourselves and listen to what the other was saying." Charles (EFT client): "Certainly I learned to listen more.... I realized when listening to a tape recorder ... that I talk too much."	
Encourage responsibility in changing their stance in the cycle	Ms. O'Neil (IFS student): "That's what we're working at—the ability to notice when it's a part and then to be able to ... see if there is enough critical mass of self either with one person or between the couple that we can have a different response in relationship to these parts instead of really letting them run the show." Tiffany (CBT client): "One of the things that my therapist would work with me on was asserting myself initially ... rather than store, store, store, and then explode, or let it magnify and then distort."	

Note. CBT, cognitive-behavioral therapy; EFT, emotionally focused therapy; IFS, internal family systems therapy.

talks, and helping each client choose how to respond. Each relational model has several interventions aimed at this end. Slowing down the process helps couples to begin to explore other possibilities for their relational difficulties. The client essentially says, "I'm willing to try something different here."

Helping Couples Stand Meta to Themselves

Once a couple has slowed down, therapists help them alter the cycle by encouraging them to stand meta to (i.e., outside of) themselves. When standing meta, a couple begins to see each partner's role in the interactional cycle and to explore other possibilities of interacting with each other. This process unfolds during several model-specific interventions, such as monitoring self-talk in cognitive-behavioral therapy (Dattilio, 2005). In this intervention, clients are encouraged to step outside themselves in an interaction and look at what they are telling themselves about their partner during an argument. A client may tell him- or herself something like "I'm starting to feel defensive because he's coming home late. I interpret his lateness to mean that he does not want to be with me, but I learned in our last therapy session that he is late really because he does not want to get verbally attacked by me." Other interventions that facilitate this goal include focusing on the "softer" intent or needs underlying "harsh" language, and helping each partner hear the other differently.

Encouraging Personal Responsibility

Once clients have slowed down their processes and can correctly perceive their roles in the interactional cycle, relational therapists help them take responsibility for changing their roles in the cycle. Clients are encouraged to take personal responsibility more by the language used by the therapist over the course of therapy rather than through interventions aimed specifically at encouraging responsibility. A phrase that encourages personal responsibility could be "So, the next time your partner starts yelling at you, you need to recognize that as her attempt to connect with you. Resist the urge to withdraw, and try to respond to what you think is underneath her anger." A response to the same situation that instead encourages passive victimization could be "My word, I can't believe how mean your partner is. No wonder you're so afraid!" If therapy consists of too much of the latter statement without much of the former, change is not likely to happen.

Additional Variables That Influence the Success of the Intervention Stage

As in the early stages of therapy, the success of the aforementioned tasks is determined largely by the safety of the therapeutic environment, the degree to which the process is repeated, the therapist's ability to present interventions in a way that is direct but does not elicit resistance, a client's willingness to accept personal responsibility for his or her role in the relationship problems and to commit to work on the relationship, and the degree to which the client trusts that the therapist is acting in his or her best interest. It is also important that the client be able to grasp psychological and systemic concepts, since standing meta to oneself and changing one's behavior as a result, for example, requires a substantial degree of cognitive complexity.

Also key to the success of the intervention stage is a *therapeutic alliance that is isomorphic to the goals of therapy*. The therapeutic relationship should serve as a model for the client relationship. Attributes that clients need to change can be modeled by the therapist in the therapeutic alliance. For example, if a client needs to stand up for him- or herself to his or her spouse more, the therapist will purposefully model that behavior by standing up to the spouse. In short, the therapeutic alliance should model the change that needs to take place.

When Luis and Alida began therapy, all they could focus on was trying to change each other. The more Sara helped Alida see Luis as stressed and overwhelmed, and Luis see Alida as lonely and frightened, however, the more they started to abandon their stance in the pursue–withdraw cycle. As each gradually started to see how his or her own stance led to the stance they disliked in their partner, they opened up to Sara's efforts to help them explore more effective ways of communicating their thoughts and feelings. Luis felt more emboldened to open up to Alida as he saw Sara communicate with Alida the same openness he feared using. Alida was able to soften her communication with Luis the more she saw how Sara's softer stance helped Luis open up the way she had always wanted him to. The more they practiced their new approach to communicating in session, the easier it became to do the same at home.

The Outcome Stage

As we mentioned earlier, different models tend to produce similar results, supporting the systemic principle of *equifinality*. In this study, more commonalities were found in the way that clients changed than in any other stage of therapy. Despite the application of diverse models of treatment, clients changed in remarkably similar ways. The two main ways in which clients in this study changed were *softening* and *making space for the other*. Again, we present these two outcomes not as a comprehensive list of the ways that couples and families change but rather as an illustration of our claim that many models lead couples and families to the same ends. These two outcomes are reached by many—though not all—couples and families.

Softening

As couple therapy successfully progresses, clients willingly abandon their previously harsh, critical view of their partner (and, in some instances, themselves) in favor of a more patient, accepting approach. When faced with an event that would have previously triggered a harsh response, angry emotions, and critical thoughts, they instead act, feel, and think more "softly." They are better able to regulate their emotions and as a result are more emotionally accessible to each other. They treat each other more kindly, feel more compassion toward each other, and give each other the benefit of the doubt more, trusting in each other's good intentions. They see their emotional needs as valid; they trust that they can own those needs and that their partner will meet them. They are able to independently exit what previously would have turned into a negative interactional cycle.

Making Space for the Other

Maturana (1992) defines "violence" as "holding an idea to be true such that another's idea is wrong and must change." Conversely, he defines "love" as "opening space for the existence of another." His definitions of "violence" and "love" provide the backdrop for common shifts experienced by clients that are successful in couple therapy. Dysfunctional interactional cycles are restrictive of personal growth. In a typical pursue–withdraw pattern, for example, the pursuer sets aside his or her patience, kindness, tolerance, and other such attributes. The withdrawer neglects his or her assertiveness. Both often lose self-confidence as their efforts to connect consistently fail to produce the desired results. As interactional cycles shift from destructive to healing, the couple abandons attempts to control in favor of supporting each other's autonomy. As each partner begins replacing his or her attempts to control the other with support for the partner's autonomy, energy is freed up for each partner to foster his or her own neglected attributes; the emotional and physical space provided by the partner allows him or her the latitude to do so.

Abandoning attempts to control each other also enables couples to "slow down" in other aspects of their life. Clients in the study reported feeling less worried, stressed, anxious, and compulsive overall. Many said that they enjoyed life in general a lot more—they laughed at more things, found meaning in helping others, and enjoyed a "deeper" life than they had before. This started to happen as they stopped trying to change things *outside* (i.e., their partner) and started to change things *inside* themselves.

As efforts to connect with each other start to succeed, each individual's confidence and self-efficacy increased. This is often true both in the marriage relationship and in other areas of the couple's life. As each person started to nurture the other's autonomy more, most clients in the study reported being more confident in their jobs, as parents, and so forth.

By 4 months into therapy Luis and Alida viewed each other completely differently. They saw the good intent behind each other's actions and felt a lot more compassion toward each other. They treated each other more kindly. Luis was amazed at how much his confidence increased as Sara helped him identify and express what he was feeling. Not only his marriage had improved as a result, but also his business was prospering as he became more assertive toward the problems he faced. And Sara helped Alida try to understand Luis before responding to him; this helped Alida feel more in control during interactions with others. The more she listened to others before responding, the more patient and understanding she became not only with Luis but also with her children, friends, and others.

As we mentioned earlier, these changes are consistent with several different models, even though they call the changes different names. Whether you call these changes becoming more securely attached (emotionally focused therapy), more differentiated (Bowen), getting parts to step back so that self can lead (internal family systems therapy), adopting a liberating narrative (narrative therapy), integrating disowned aspects of the self (object relations therapy), or any number of similar model-specific descriptions of these phenomena, the changes are still the same, and they are achieved through pragmatically similar yet conceptually different pathways.

Strengths and Limitations

We believe that our model can help clinicians do better therapy. Our model provides a list of broad and narrow pantheoretical variables for clinicians to track as their clients progress through therapy. Our model provides numerous questions a clinician could ask about the process of therapy if it becomes stuck (see Chapter 12, pp. 176–177, for a list of these questions). Moreover, if a client is not responding well to a therapist's approach, our model can make the leap to a different approach feel much less daunting since our model orients the therapist to similar processes and points to similar ends regardless of what model is being used.

This model represents the first efforts that we are aware of to combine broad and narrow common factors into a coherent meta-model describing how change occurs in couple therapy. As with all research, there are limitations inherent in the research design that limit the generalizability of the findings. First of all, the model is not inclusive of all factors that affect therapy. For example, we did not explicitly investigate larger contextual factors such as race, gender, and sociopolitical contexts. Future research integrating these factors into the model could make it more comprehensive. In the meantime, however, we think that a culturally sensitive therapist would not have difficulty adapting our model to fit a diverse clientele.

Furthermore, all we know is that the variables mentioned occurred—not whether or not they are statistically related to outcome. That will hopefully be determined by future research. Furthermore, even though standard precautions were taken to minimize researcher bias, there are undoubtedly aspects of therapy that were missed, or, conversely, overemphasized simply because of researcher biases. Despite these limitations, we believe that it is a useful model that is broad enough to allow for use by diverse therapists and models and yet specific enough to provide clinical, research, and training guidance. We hope that testing, expansion, and refinement of the model will continue.

Special Considerations for Family Therapy

This meta-model was designed specifically for couple therapy, but we believe that it can find use in family therapy as well. Nevertheless, we believe that there are important contraindications when using this

meta-model as a guide for family therapy. First, couple therapy generally assumes equal responsibility for change except in cases where an
imbalance of power exists such as domestic violence or, as many femi-
nist scholars claim, nonegalitarian marriages (Murphy & Eckhardt,
2005). Family therapy typically does not assume equal responsibility
for change due to the power imbalance inherent in a parent–child relationship. When both parents and children need to change, the duty
to take the first step centers on the parents. Second, many effective
family therapy models incorporate larger systems into treatment—
schools, churches, community resources, and so forth (Doherty &
Beaton, 2000; Fraenkel, 2006). The couple therapy model we outline
offers little guidance in that regard.

Despite the meta-model's limitations when applied to families, it
overlaps with established family therapy models such as functional
family therapy (Sexton & Alexander, 2005) in that it emphasizes the
importance of engagement and motivation during the early stages
of therapy and provides related guidance for those. The principles
guiding the client's adoption of a therapist's model as outlined in this
study would likely apply to family therapy as well. Furthermore, since
most established family therapy models are systemic, the principles
guiding the use of interactional cycles as a conceptual and interventive tool, as outlined in this model, could find use in family therapy as
well. Similarly, the common outcomes achieved in this study are likely
to also be worthy goals in family therapy.

10

The Case against Common Factors

The common factors perspective we have described makes intuitive sense, is continually confirmed in clinical settings, and is strongly supported by research—and yet this view of treatment also has vociferous critics. In this chapter we look at such criticisms and present our responses to them.

In launching this discussion, it is crucial to highlight that very few critics (and among them only the most extreme outliers who are prepared to distort the existing data) suggest that common factors are unimportant. Most critics of common factors accept that such aspects of treatment as the therapeutic relationship and the generation of hope do make a difference (Chambless, 2002; Sexton, Gilman, & Johnson-Erickson, 2005). Instead, they aim their criticism primarily at the most radical of common factor viewpoints, such as those of Wampold (2001) or Duncan, Miller, and colleagues (Hubble et al., 1999). These radical common factor approaches suggest that psychotherapy *is* the application of common factors, treatment approaches are irrelevant to outcome, and efforts to hone treatment approaches are misguided exercises.

Even though we have great respect for the work of such scholars as Wampold, Hubble, Duncan, and Miller and want to acknowledge their significant contributions to our work, as we have highlighted in this volume, our own approach is significantly different. In contrast to their more extreme position, we view the common factors in couple and family therapy as the most crucial ingredients in treatment but not the only relevant ingredients. Nonetheless, there remains a considerable gap between the critics of common factor approaches and our own position. The typical critics of common factors suggest that specific treatments play a far more important role in treatment effectiveness than we are suggesting in this volume (Chambless, 2002; Sexton et al., 2004). We discuss each of the key criticisms they offer of common factors in considerable detail in turn.

• *Criticism 1: There are hundreds of studies that show that specific treatments are superior to alternative treatments.* There is a very different way of looking at family therapy, and more generally at psychotherapy, than that described in this volume. This is the viewpoint of the empirically supported psychotherapies (ESTs; sometimes referred to as "empirically validated psychotherapies"). The EST viewpoint originated with the adaptation of medication trials to the study of psychotherapy (Westen et al., 2004). In testing the safety and effectiveness of medication, an experimental design called the randomized clinical trial is utilized to find whether medications work as well or better than those already established and better than a placebo. In this design, subjects are all put in a pool and randomly assigned to the groups receiving various medications and the placebo. Then, the groups are compared in their functioning after the treatment. Treatments that do better than the placebo and equally well as or better than other well-established treatments come to be identified as effective.

Proponents of ESTs suggest that the same methods should be utilized to test the impact of treatments—and that treatments do have a differential impact. This cadre of scientists has had only modest impact in the world of clinicians and clinical settings, but it does have enormous influence in such government agencies as the NIMH in the United States and other similar groups around the globe and increasing influence with third-party payers. In studies used to establish ESTs, randomized potential clients are assigned to different psychotherapies or, more typically, psychotherapy and no treatment or a placebo treatment, and the differences between groups are assessed. The standard (also cited in Chapter 5) most frequently invoked for suggesting a treatment has achieved the status of an EST (Chambless, 1999) is that there be at least two high-quality randomized clinical trials that confirm the impact of the treatment on a specific disorder, with these studies being conducted by at least two different investigators (so that one person alone cannot be the source for research confirming an EST, thereby limiting the possibility of biased reporting and allegiance effects).

ESTs have begun to appear in couple and family therapies. For treating marital distress, popular ESTs include emotionally focused couple therapy (Johnson, 2003b), behavioral marital therapy (Jacobson, 1980), and integrative behavioral couple therapy (Christensen et al., 2004). For treating adolescent delinquency, conduct disorder, and substance use disorder, ESTs include brief strategic family therapy (Santisteban et al., 2003), multisystemic therapy (Henggeler, Schoenwald, Borduin, Rowland, & Cunningham, 1998), multidimensional family therapy (Liddle et al., 2005), functional family therapy (Sexton & Alexander, 2003), and multidimesional treatment foster care (Chamberlain & Smith, 2005). For treating severe mental illness, ESTs include family psychoeducation skill-building treatments for schizophrenia (Anderson et al., 1980; Falloon, 2002) and bipolar disorder (Miklowitz et al., 2000, 2003). Certainly, each of these treatments is a carefully constructed, well-considered treatment. Considerable time and effort have gone into the development of each therapy (as is true for many treatments). And each has been supported by more than one clinical trial and become widely disseminated around the world. Such care and research in treatment development seems to us admirable, but we become concerned when proponents of these ESTs go further than praising these treatments, arguing that such treatments are clearly superior to others since they have been established as effective while the impact of other treatments remains in doubt, and therefore their preferred EST become the treatment of first choice.

As we emphasized in Chapter 5, establishing a treatment as an EST or what Shadish and Baldwin (2003) have called an MAST (a meta-analytically supported treatment) has considerable value as long as one recognizes the limitations of these designations. The moderate common factors position acknowledges that randomized clinical trials are necessary to prove to external audiences (such as governments, third-party payers, and other social scientists) that our treatments are efficacious. We also have suggested that there is merit to any model's demonstrating that it is efficacious. The research in support of ESTs and MASTs has also added other value in allowing for secondary analyses of such aspects of treatment as the impact of the alliance that certainly would never be funded in today's medical model-driven funded research environment.

And yet, it is fairly easy for the designation of a treatment as an EST to appear to reveal more than it actually does. There are a number of reasons for this. First, there are basic questions about whether this method of deciding which treatments are most effective is applicable to psychotherapy in the way it works for drug research. We also question whether it is the best method for assessing psychotherapy if not supplemented by other approaches. Bear in mind that medication trials contrast drugs and the placebo, which generally are fairly easy to present in a way that the subjects don't know to which group they have been assigned (though even here the argument is sometimes made that subjects do in fact figure out which is the placebo fairly readily by the presence or absence of side effects). Psychotherapies are very difficult to "blind" (subjects usually know whether they are in the control group) and virtually impossible to double-blind since the therapist virtually always knows the group to which he or she is assigned. Furthermore, even the notion of "placebo" is problematic in psychotherapy research since nonspecific factors play an important role in experimental as well as control groups. Finally, in drug treatment, who delivers the treatment is much less important than in psychotherapy, where who delivers the treatment is often crucial.

Further, there are innumerable problems in creating an effective design to test for efficacy even in the best studies. For example, those who fit into a protocol for research are normally quite different than typical clients who present with a range of difficulties including the problem in question. In typical EST research the presence of such "comorbidities" (the term used in the context of the medical model) causes such clients to be excluded from the research. For these clients, comorbid problems beyond the one in focus in the study typically have been ruled out as absent.

Therapists also are rarely as skillful in two different approaches when treatments are compared, and the number of therapists involved in these research projects typically is small. That leaves much of the impact of the various treatments vulnerable to how well each therapist manifests common factors (therapists assigned to different groups may differ in their abilities to do so) as well as his or her ability to implement the specific treatment delivered. Indeed, one argument that has been made about the most prominent EST psychotherapy study, the NIMH collaborative treatment of depression study (Elkin, 1994), was that the differences among groups were largely due to the differential effectiveness of a couple of the therapists in their ability to work with clients (Elkin, 1999). As noted in Chapter 4, there was compelling evidence in this study that therapist effects were highly significant but treatment effects were not.

Further, treatments are typically studied in clients who share a diagnosis in fairly small samples that rarely are representative of the diversity in the general population. This leaves open the distinct possibility that the effects would be different in clients from, for example, another culture or age group. ESTs gain their legitimacy through efficacy studies with tight controls for internal validity (that is, whether the method allows for the demonstration that the treatment is effective in the sample) and that typically say little about external validity (that is, whether the treatment would work with others who differ in substantial ways). Other methodological problems limiting these studies include the difficulties presented by clients dropping out (the treatment may be effective among those completing the treatment, but many clients may not do so) and the intrinsic need to limit the length of the treatment to that of a medication trial due cost considerations (thus, causing the treatment to be structured in relation to the needs of research rather than the best length of treatment for the problem). Perhaps most of all, this body of work has been criticized for its selection of the specific treatments to be studied (creating the possibility of becoming an EST) because treatments that have proven effective in treating one problem almost always need to obtain separate funding for treating another problem (thus creating a circular problem, that is, leading to ESTs today largely being versions of cognitive-behavioral therapy).

Additionally, the impact of these treatments is not as clear as typically presented. Treatments are typically compared to no treatment or the infamous "treatment-as-usual" in systems that offer little treatment or even problematic treatments (such as incarceration for adolescent problems). Sometimes these "treatment-as-usual" therapies are disorganized "seat-of-the-pants" interventions offered by well-meaning but overextended practitioners. As noted in Chapter 4, the very fact that an intervention is well organized and coherent (independent of specific interventions) may make it more effective than a disorganized alternative. Treatment-as-usual therapists are also often less committed than their counterparts in favored "experimental" conditions. Other studies have contrasted a treatment under study with a sham version of psychotherapy, bearing no real resemblance to what actual clinicians do. As Drew Westen and colleagues (Westen, Stirman, & DeRubeis, 2006) have put it:

> If researchers want clinicians to take their research seriously, they will need to take clinicians seriously. That is, they will need to compare their treatments to treatments as practiced by experienced well-paid professionals in private practice, not to no treatment, waitlist controls, worst practice labeled TAU (i.e., treatment by

overworked, often undereducated therapists in underfunded settings), or intent-to-fail conditions (e.g., "supportive" therapy with
no theoretical goals carried out by graduate students who know
they are in the non-bona fide treatment condition. (p. 171)

There are only a few studies that truly compare ESTs with other widely
practiced treatments or other ESTs. This leaves the distinct possibility
that all bone fide widely accepted treatments might well emerge as
ESTs if studied. Most treatments simply aren't studied.

A case in point can readily be made in the individual treatment
of depression. Because all of the initial treatment studies focused on
cognitive-behavioral treatments for depression, at one time the only
ESTs were all cognitive-behavioral treatments. Then, through some
lobbying at NIMH, a psychodynamic treatment, interpersonal psychotherapy, was developed and validated (Elkin, 1994; Klerman,
Weissman, Rounsaville, & Chevron, 1995). And subsequently, Les
Greenberg and colleagues showed that the quite distinct experiential
emotionally focused therapy was also effective (Elliott, Watson, Goldman, & Greenberg, 2004), as Neil Jacobson demonstrated as well
with a couple therapy (albeit a cognitive-behavioral one; Jacobson et
al., 1991). Had the later two groups not emerged, all ESTs for depression would involve individual cognitive-behavioral therapy. The types
of approaches that become ESTs are clearly closely correlated with
the various alternatives that are investigated.

There also are powerful allegiance effects in the studies of these
treatments. Treatments almost inevitably do better that are the preferred treatments of the investigators. In fact, one meta-analysis found
this factor to be the single most important one in determining the
outcome of a treatment study (Luborsky et al., 1999). As we noted
in Chapter 4, Wampold (2001) offers compelling empirical evidence
that allegiance effects account for more of the outcome variance in
psychotherapy than do treatment effects.

To return to our thesis, for the majority of problems clearly the
common factors across treatments are more salient than the differences across couple and family therapies. Therapists all form alliances,
engage hope, set goals, and engage the other common factors we have
discussed. The research indicates that only a small percentage of the
impact of any treatment can be attributed to the treatment stripped of
its common factor attributes.

This conclusion is overwhelmingly the case where treatments aim
at broad issues in living such as feeling better, finding meaning in

life, enjoying relationships, or doing better at work. Note that none of these goals is ever the focal point of an EST, which—given the paradigm derived from NIMH studies of medication—only zeroes in on problems formulated within the phenomenology of the DSM of the American Psychiatric Association. Additionally, even assuming a medical model perspective focused on the treatment of syndromes as labeled in DSM, many problems such as dysthymic disorder or generalized anxiety disorder or adjustment disorder clearly are broadly regarded by clinicians as amenable to a broad range of methods of treatment. And here each treatment that has come to be tested has proven effective (Greenberg & Watson, 1998; Jacobson et al., 1991; Klerman & Weissman, 1991; Westen et al., 2004). It always is also essential to remember that there has yet to be an approach that has proven ineffective in research in treating such problems (Westen et al., 2004).

In fairness to those who support ESTs, it is our opinion (as noted earlier) that there are treatments that do appear to be uniquely effective for certain highly specialized problems. There are problems for which typical clinicians clearly recognize the difficulty in treating populations with these difficulties and ESTs specifically designed to be effective with these problems. Examples include panic disorder (Craske & Barlow, 2008), obsessive–compulsive disorder (Franklin & Foa, 2007), severe marital distress (Christensen et al., 2004), borderline personality disorder (Koerner & Linehan, 2002), and adolescent externalizing disorders (Pickrel & Henggeler, 1996). Although some clinicians might claim broad effectiveness with every problem, there does seem a place for highly specialized treatments for such problems. However, it should be emphasized that clients manifesting such problems clearly make up only a small minority of all clients. Further, as multiple similar ESTs are developed for treating these problems, it also seems clear (as we pointed out in Chapter 5) that there is often not one unique effective treatment for such problems but rather a class of effective treatments that share core characteristics.

Let us cite some examples among family therapies. It seems clear that conjoint treatments are vastly superior to individual treatments for couple distress and that emotionally focused couple therapy, behavioral couple therapy, and integrative behavioral couple therapy have considerable impact on severe marital difficulties (Gurman, 1978; Jacobson et al., 2000; Johnson, 2003a). Nonetheless, it seems likely that a range of methods of couple therapy that cover similar territory are likely ultimately to prove effective. Similarly, multisystemic treatments that include work with family and individual teenagers in intense treatments appear to be treatments of choice for the range of acting-out and substance use problems in adolescents (Kazdin, 2007). A half-dozen similar treatments differing in their methods but involving a systems perspective, treatment intensity, assertive methods of treatment engagement, and typically some individual focus on the teenager all have proved effective (Henggeler et al., 1998; Liddle et al., 2005; Robbins et al., 2003; Sexton & Alexander, 2005). A third example can be found in treatments that combine medication, individual help for clients, and help with the family in treating the more severe forms of mental disorder such as schizophrenia or bipolar disorder (Anderson et al., 1980; Falloon, 1993; Miklowitz, 2008; Rea et al., 2003). These are clearly effective therapies in the context of difficult-to-treat problems. However, we also caution that there remains no reason to believe that other treatments that include these broad factors in each of these specific contexts would be any less effective than the trademarked therapies for treating these problems. New therapies incorporating similar elements enter the lists of ESTs at regular intervals, and indeed at the National Institute of Mental Health and National Institute of Drug Abuse there are in process some tests of several "new" treatments that relate to slightly different methods but similar approaches for dealing with each of these difficulties.

So, in sum, ESTs, while valuable, have their limitations that are not always acknowledged when clinical scientists refer to them as the "gold standard." They are invaluable in establishing efficacy and credibility with external audiences, and they have special relevance when treating certain hard-to-treat problems. Furthermore, as we noted in Chapter 5, there is nothing inherent in the methodology of randomized clinical trials that would prevent the study of common factors from being undertaken within these investigations. However, it is also unfortunate that other types of research, such as progress research (which examines the effects of a typical therapy session by session as it unfolds) (Pinsof & Wynne, 2000) or research on how to better engage common factors are not widely supported by funding agencies. Those kinds of research would likely provide better information for learning how and why therapy is effective than clinical trials to establish treatment efficacy.

• *Criticism 2: The empirical support of common factors arises from meta-analysis, which is not a sufficiently nuanced approach to fully reflect the impact of treatment factors.* This criticism principally comes from those who think of the clinical trial (despite the problems we have described with it) as the gold standard of research and will not accept other forms of evidence as germane to a research question. They consider anything other than a tightly controlled clinical trial questionable evidence.

Clearly, summative approaches such as meta-analyses are crucial to the study of common factors. Although clinical trial designs can be used to study the impact of common factors in secondary analysis (for example, to analyze the relative effectiveness an impact of different therapists in the study), one simply cannot experimentally manipulate common factors to make them the primary focus of a clinical trial. Stated most bluntly, you cannot randomly assign therapists to do bad therapy.

For example, picture this hypothetical research study. An investigator proposes a study that contrasts clients receiving a treatment that encourages high levels of therapeutic alliance and the engagement of hope with clients whose treatment is deliberately designed to be rated low in these qualities. That research would *never* get through the review of an institution or university research review committee precisely because it is almost universally accepted among mental health professionals that these two factors *do* matter in treatment and therefore clients receiving treatment without them are inherently receiving inferior treatment. So, the institutional review board that oversees the research would not find being in the control group a safe option for those assigned to it—which is simultaneously a testimony to the vital importance of common factors but yet also a constraint to their becoming the direct focus of clinical trial research.

As with the use of certain elements in medicine that predate the experimental method, it is an assumption of "common practice" that common factors do matter. In medicine and most activities, common practice is regarded as applicable until disconfirmed by research.

Furthermore, to our knowledge, there is no existing research to support the thesis that common factors do not matter. The only even marginally relevant data utilized to challenge the impact of common factors consists of a number of studies already described by us that show that carefully honed treatments work better than pseudotreatments that consist of unfocused bland support. However, as we have stressed, this group of studies falls short of being an exemplary version of a common factor approach such as the one we subscribe to in this volume. Further, common factors are not "islands unto themselves" but rather work *through* the treatment methods (Sprenkle &

Blow, 2004b). In fact, it would be difficult to tease out what was pro-
ducing the effects of the carefully honed experimental treatment since
common factors are inextricably embedded into it. Can you imagine,
say, delivering an intervention without developing a therapeutic alliance or not using other non-model-specific aspects of being a good
therapist? As we emphasized in Chapter 1 as well as earlier in this
chapter, the whole notion of "placebo controls" breaks down for psychotherapy research since it is impossible not to have common factors
present in both treatment *and* control groups.

    With this in mind, we return to the criticism that the research
evidence for the importance of common factors derives primarily
from meta-analysis and the suggestion that the evidence is weak or
debatable. It certainly is true that because the random assignment of
clients to therapists who produce low amounts of common factors is
ethically inappropriate, the principal evidence for common factors
does come from correlational and meditational analyses, typically
presented in meta-analyses, assessing differences in outcome between
those high and low in common factors within treatment groups. These
results have been summarized in several prominent literature reviews
(Lambert & Bergin, 1994; Lambert & Hill, 1994; Lambert & Ogles,
2004) and meta-analyses (Kazdin, 2003; Shadish & Baldwin, 2002,
2003; Shadish et al., 1993; Wampold, 2001; Wampold, Minami, Tierney, Baskin, & Bhati, 2005; Wampold et al., 1997). In each of these
reviews and meta-analyses, common factors emerge as important
sources of variance—in fact, always more important than treatment
factors. The only real debate is about the extent of the impact of common factors and treatment factors, and how much more important
common factors are than treatment factors. The arguments about
these data range from those suggesting treatment factors having virtually no impact (Hubble et al., 1999), to those suggesting some degree
of impact (Orlinsky, Grawe, & Parks, 1994),[1] to those arguing for
higher impact (Chambless & Ollendick, 2001; Sexton et al., 2004)
Thus, there is almost no argument about the direction of the findings
of these literature reviews or meta-analyses.

    Admittedly, there *are* problems with meta-analysis. Critics argue
that meta-analyses remain susceptible to the inclusion of methodologically weak studies that could affect the findings. Meta-analyses are
only as good as the studies they meta-analyze. Perhaps many poor

---

[1]Of course, "specific factors" scholars would rate the impact of treatment factors as high
(Chambless, 2002; Sexton & Ridley, 2004) as well.

therapies have been studied that reduce the effect of treatment factors overall as compared to common factors, or perhaps the effects of treatment only emerge in the best studies. Yet, such criticisms appear to us to have been addressed though results that have demonstrated that the methodological quality of the research, the specific problem area, or the kind of treatment studied does not seem to impact the finding. Virtually every meta-analysis shows a vital role for common factors and several have demonstrated that this finding is as powerful in the best of studies as in all the studies (Shadish & Baldwin, 2002; Smith & Glass, 1977). The findings in support of the importance of common factors in meta-analysis are consistent across efforts in a way that would be unlikely if weaker studies were causing the effect. Lest this be taken as a problem of statistical analysis, it is important to emphasize that careful literature reviews with an eye to the quality of research have confirmed the findings of these meta-analyses (Lambert, 2004; Norcross, 2002b).

Other criticisms of the meta-analyses in support of the importance of common factors relative to treatment factors have been based on misunderstandings of these analyses. For example, Sexton et al. (2004) argued that meta-analyses have only compared loosely defined or diffuse "schools" of therapy that are juxtaposed against specific treatment models. In point of fact, however, both Wampold (2001) and Luborsky (Luborsky et al., 2002) limited their meta-analyses to comparisons among only bona fide treatments. Similarly, Sexton et al. (2004) argued that some meta-analyses were small (few studies summarized) and therefore there was inadequate statistical power to show differences among treatments. However, in meta-analyses the standard errors are much smaller since each study estimate is based on the study's number of participants. Therefore, if three studies are aggregated, each with an N of 20, it would be similar to a study of 60 participants, not three (Sprenkle & Blow, 2004b).

It is certainly possible that, as the technique of meta-analysis becomes more refined and meta-analysts are able to do more fine-grained coding (e.g., isolating types of problems or types of clients), more evidence for treatment specificity may emerge. However, we think it highly unlikely that any well-done meta-analysis will ever demonstrate that specific treatment factors are more potent than common factors. In fact, we believe that one of the most robust data-based findings in all of psychotherapy research is that the largest portion of outcome variance is attributable to mechanisms of change that are common to all successful treatments (Sprenkle & Blow, 2004b).

• *Criticism 3: Common factors advocacy is an either–or position in that it denigrates treatment models and empirically supported models and it oversimplifies the process of change.* This set of arguments aims at the exaggerated view of common factors in family therapy and more generally in psychotherapy. We do see merit in this position if limited to that exaggerated viewpoint. To suggest that it does not matter at all how therapists conceptualize and intervene is a head-in-the-sand position that we trust we have roundly repudiated in this volume. We have all seen well-meaning therapists in their first meetings with families who readily show caring but fail to engage the family because they lack a coherent plan for helping the family. The field of family therapy is filled with models developed over many years that present thoughtful ways of engaging and helping with problems and are well worth learning.

The argument for attributing greater importance to treatment factors is much stronger than the one diminishing the importance of common factors. An incredible amount of work has gone into the development of treatments, be they the newer EST variety or the old-fashioned approach. These models have evolved over the past 100 years in psychotherapy and 60 years in family therapy to become more and more sophisticated in engaging methods that help change human behavior. Today's approaches are filled with effective strategies for change and what is now a huge toolkit of interventions that have great value. Furthermore, models are typically based on theories of personality and psychopathology that provide insight into human functioning and often provide a helpful perspective about what is important in life (e.g. authenticity, autonomy, connection, collaboration, feeling emotion, optimism, reason, knowledge about self, being symptom-free, mindfulness). Although these ideas may not represent universal truths for all, such core values at the heart of treatment models create potential helpful directions for changing one's life. Further, they help us as clinicians see problems in a clear-cut way that enables intervention. When a family enters treatment for a problem such as an adolescent's substance use, there inevitably are innumerable factors that could become the focus of intervention. Treatment models help the therapist to sort through this information and suggest a path toward change. Models also clearly help in the development of psychotherapists. As one of us has written elsewhere (Lebow, 2002), new therapists typically become lost without the road path of a clear model of practice.

Thus, we do not mean to denigrate treatments. They are, after all, one of the best ways of generating some of the common factors such as hope and alliance that we describe in this book. We merely pause at the point where they become what one of us has called "sacred" (Sprenkle & Blow, 2004a), reified as the *best* or *only* path toward change. Treatments invoke change processes that almost always can also be invoked as well by other treatments. They represent one useful way of seeing the world that can help people change—but not the only one. And each model has better applicability to certain types of human situations than others. We have also stressed the value of empirically supported treatments.

However, we believe that moving away from the tradition of competing models both in research and dialogue (as exemplified in the clinical trial horse race between approaches) and toward understanding the common shared ground of methods of practice and tools that can enable all clinical practice will prove more productive than continuing such debates and horse races. For example, the newer research tradition called "progress research"—looking at how clients progress over the ongoing course of treatment and providing feedback to clinicians about treatment progress as treatment advances—seems to us far more valuable for learning about clients and helping them (Howard et al., 1996; Pinsof & Wynne, 2000) than a primary focus on distal treatment outcomes in highly controlled clinical trial research centered on disorders. Progress research looks at client functioning and alliance on a session-by-session basis and can immeasurably add to the client's treatment by providing ongoing feedback and accountability about how the treatment is progressing. Michael Lambert and his colleagues (Lambert, Harmon, Slade, Whipple, & Hawkins, 2005) have reported on a series of studies in which therapists (regardless of their preferred treatment method) improved significantly when they were given session-by-session feedback regarding short-term progress. While still keeping an eye on long-term goals, this approach encourages changing aspects of the treatment when progress is less than expected. This approach focuses less on how to treat a particular diagnostic problem and more on understanding what the keys to helping the client truly are, and then addressing those issues— what Pinsof (1995) calls the problem maintenance structure. Pinsof and colleagues (Pinsof & Lebow, 2005; Pinsof & Wynne, 2000) have recently developed a system for assessing progress in couple and family therapy consisting of a set of scales (the systemic therapy inventory of change) and a highly sophisticated computer feedback system for tracking client progress. Research methods such as progress research are emerging in psychotherapy research that seem much more likely to be fruitful than the accent on finding the most efficacious treatment matched to the disorder via clinical trial research.

Drew Westen (Westen et al., 2004) points to a client who was depressed and had sexual problems. ESTs for depression or sexual problems would have pointed to structured ways for overcoming these problems, typically through changing his self-talk. Yet, this client had those problems primarily because of unaddressed issues relating to his sexual identity. As the client came to terms with being gay, the depression and sexual problems subsided. For such a case, an EST would simply miss the essence of the problem—precisely because the problem is almost always formulated in terms of a diagnostic category defined in terms of the medical model. The vast majority of clients do not neatly fit into such simple categories.

We need to move discussions of common factors away from the straw man argument often invoked against proponents that "treatments do not matter at all." The framework we bring to this book allows room for learning from specific treatments and even for applying special interventions in certain specific situations. However, we strongly believe that it is more valuable for couple and family therapists to find ways to maximize their abilities to enhance common factors than to focus on learning new treatments just because they are designated ESTs (Lebow, 1987). Assuming an active stance on the part of the therapist and a bona fide set of methods of intervention that are brought to the clients, what goes on between therapist and client is far more important than whether the treatment is one of the ESTs. Ultimately, we believe that a set of principles for practice is likely to emerge within couple and family therapy (for example, teaching communication skills to clients is helpful whenever theirs are deficient), but such a set of principles is far removed from the prescriptive regimens of most ESTs. It is striking to note that one of the most popularly supported ESTs in family therapy, multisystemic therapy for adolescent substance abuse and delinquency (Henggeler & Lee, 2003), primarily sets its focus on which system is most important to work within (family, school, peer, etc.), a quite broad level for determining intervention. In looking at the state of treatment in family therapy, and even at the direction of the development of the most sophisticated ESTs, it seems to us that building treatment solidly on the foundation of common factors and bringing to bear a range of relevant and effective intervention strategies applicable to the case at hand (Lebow, 1997; Pinsof, 1995) represents the future direction of the field.

Our approach may not have the marketing appeal of today's hottest and best validated treatment model (as the brochures often describe ESTs). However, we believe it speaks far better to the accumulated wisdom in our field that has evolved over several decades. Bringing evidence to bear is essential to the development of practice. It helps separate the theories, strategies, and techniques that have value from those that do not; moreover, it helps us to understand when and under what circumstances particular methods are helpful, allowing evidence to appropriately inform practice. However, considering evidence assessing the impact of treatment to be important does not necessitate buying into the notion that these narrowly defined evidence-based treatments are necessarily *the* best methods of practice. It seems obvious to us that ultimately therapies have their impact by engaging core human processes that move toward change and that common factors are typically the key elements that engage these core human processes. And rather than the profession's moving in the direction of experts trained in one or two of what will soon be hundreds of ESTs, we would do far better to rely on common factors and other principles of change that underlie methods that seem to work particularly well with specific groups of people (Castonguay & Beutler, 2006a).

11

Common Factors Training and Supervision

As we mentioned earlier, the three of us are clinicians, educators, and supervisors. The question "What makes a therapist effective?" is of profound interest to our development as clinicians. Our answers to this question have been the focus of the majority of the book up to this point. As educators and supervisors, we are also interested in the training implications of our new paradigm. How can an educator help trainees learn therapy according to our common-factors-driven change paradigm as opposed to the predominant model-driven change paradigm? What are the benefits of our training and supervisory approaches? This chapter focuses on answering these two questions.

In Chapter 8, we discussed our belief that different relational therapy models focus on similar relational processes and have similar intervention process goals, yet their conceptualization of those processes varies widely. The assumption behind comparative efficacy research has been that one of these conceptualizations—and the interventions that logically flow from them—is superior to all of the others (Lambert & Ogles, 2004). However, this assumption has consistently been shown to be false (Shadish & Baldwin, 2002). So, what is to be made of all the different couple and family therapy models? Is such a proliferation of models necessary, or does it make the daunting task of mastering couple and family therapy even more challenging?

We believe that having several different well-developed relational therapy models is an inevitable consequence of having so many diverse practitioners, researchers, and theoreticians. On the one hand, since there are so many widely varying beliefs, preferences, personalities, and so forth among therapists, having a variety of couple and family therapy models is a good thing. Such diversity helps ensure that a therapist can find a model or models that are a good fit with him or her as well as his or her clients—an important element of effective therapy (Blow, Davis, & Sprenkle, in press).

On the other hand, staring at a lengthy list of seemingly different relational approaches can make the task of finding an approach that is a good fit—let alone mastering any of them—seem daunting to a beginning therapist. The model-driven change approach can unwittingly add to a beleaguered trainee's dilemma by sending the message that a model can only be mastered in isolation from other models—that if you choose to master one model, by definition you are choosing *not* to master others. Although we do not think that this approach is necessarily harmful (it is better to master one model than none, right?), we do believe that it is unnecessarily limiting. Historically, model developers have argued that students should learn specific models in order to be effective, while common factors researchers often eschew the teaching of models in favor of learning broad common factors such as building the therapeutic alliance, instilling hope, and so forth (Hubble et al., 1999). These either–or stances have kept both sides locked in contentious struggles for some time, creating what we see as an artificial divide between equally important aspects of effective treatment. By invoking broad common factors *and* commonalities across models, our both–and common-factors-driven change approach can greatly simplify training.

As we mentioned in the introduction, our common-factors-driven change paradigm does not so much represent a new model of therapy as it does a new way of looking at existing models. Our training approach to learning common factors does not require educators to dramatically overhaul the content they teach, but it does have implications for the way models and other therapeutic skills are taught *in relation to one another.*

Ethan's first supervisor, Mark, was a cognitive-behavioral couple therapist. Mark encouraged Ethan to master the cognitive-behavioral model of couple therapy, as it was one of the most empirically supported treatments for marital therapy available. Ethan went along with this even though cognitive-behavioral therapy did not fit his style as well as he thought other models might. Ethan's next supervisor was a proponent of the Mental Research Institute approach and encouraged Ethan to master Mental Research Institute therapy as Mark had encouraged Ethan to master the cognitive-behavioral approach. As his program progressed, it seemed to Ethan that he was pulled from one approach to another just as he was starting to get fully familiar with it. He spent a good portion of his program thinking that he was familiar with many models but master of none. The models were all starting to blur together, and he still didn't feel as though he had a coherent approach to therapy. He was starting to get discouraged.

As Ethan began to study models more closely, he began to see several areas of overlap, both in terms of the way different models conceptualized the problems involved in relationships and in the end result that therapists strove to help clients reach. He also noticed that the interventions utilized in various models shared similar themes. Some helped clients to change the ways they related to each other, others changed the ways they thought about each other, while still others changed the ways clients felt toward each other. Ethan's confusion abated once he saw models as more similar than different. Ethan realized that he could master two widely varying approaches because they were not as different as his supervisors had claimed that they were. Ethan realized that he didn't have to start from ground zero every time he wanted to learn a new approach. Once he learned this, he mastered several approaches and felt comfortable using client feedback to use one purely throughout the entire course of treatment, to switch between different treatment models throughout treatment, or to integrate several models into an approach that fit his clients.

Assumptions Underlying Common-Factors-Driven and Model-Driven Change Training Approaches

Clients and Therapists: Who Should Be Adapting to Whom?

The importance of ensuring a fit between the therapist's model and clients' preferences is well documented in the research (Johnson & Talitman, 1997; Muir et al., 2004). The model-driven change approach requires that the client fit the therapist rather than the other way around. If all the therapist has is a hammer, he or she must turn each client into a nail before treatment can proceed. "Clients should not have to add 'figure out how to adapt to my therapist' to their already lengthy list of challenges" (Blow et al., 2007, p. 310). We also reviewed research in Chapter 4 suggesting that therapists need to adapt their levels of directiveness to client preferences and may also need to increase the level of emotional arousal of some clients while decreasing this arousal in others to keep the level moderate. We also reviewed impressive research that suggests which clients benefit from insight-oriented approaches and which respond better to skill-building and symptom-focused methods.

Most couple and family therapy models are integrative by nature and as such were developed by people who were intimately familiar with several different models and were creative enough to see the limitations of those models and come up with a new model to address those limitations. It is ironic, then, when the same model developers turn around and claim—either overtly or covertly—that their model is the only model that a clinician needs to master. It is even more unfortunate when educators—perhaps unwittingly—reinforce that paradigm by encouraging the mastery of only one model. Nobody would choose to go to a doctor that only prescribed one medication. Similarly, "No one model is so comprehensive that it precludes mastery of another" (Blow et al., 2007, p. 310).

Conversely, our common factors training approach suggests that the more models a therapist knows well, the more he or she will be able to flexibly adapt to the client's preferences. Since models are largely linguistically different ways of conceptualizing the same relational processes, a student can be trained to recognize common processes of relational distress and health (Gottman & Notarious, 2000) and the ways in which each model describes these processes. A focus would also be on the aspects of those processes most amenable to change and the common ways in which model specific interventions achieve that change (see Chapter 8 for additional elaboration). Students would be encouraged to become passionate about *theory* rather than passionate about *a theory* (Blow et al., 2007).

An Appreciation for Human Diversity Issues

When considering the fit between a model of therapy and clients, it is imperative to take into consideration human diversity issues such as culture, gender, ethnicity, sexual orientation, religion, and so forth. Some researchers assert that certain models are likely better suited for some cultures, genders, and ethnicities than others (McGoldrick, Giordano, & Garcia-Preto, 2005). Whether or not a model "works" is more complicated than seeing whether or not marital distress scores drop or a couple stops fighting. Ethical and moral issues such as sensitivity to issues of diversity and the propensity of the model to reinforce harmful stereotypes should also be taken into account when evaluating the usefulness of a model. For example, does a model encourage the therapist to value the experiences of each family member equally? Is the model flexible enough to be applicable to diverse cultures? Answers to these questions are equally as important when evaluating the usefulness of a model as are answers related to efficacy.

Underestimating Client Resourcefulness

Teaching a model as if it is the only model that will help a client improve sends a subtle (even if inadvertent) message that clients are so inept that we have to craft things just right in order for them to make use of therapy. Truthfully, though, how many times have your clients credited their change in part to something you either never said or they misunderstood? That has happened to us more times that we care to remember—some of our best therapy has been therapy that we have never actually done! It appears sometimes as though clients improve *despite* our best efforts! We are not saying that therapy is of no value. On the contrary, research suggests that most people who go to therapy improve far more than those who do not (Shadish & Baldwin, 2002). Rather, we are saying that overemphasizing the importance of any one therapeutic model underestimates a client's ability to, within reason, take what we give them and make productive use of it (Tallman & Bohart, 1999). Our approach acknowledges that fact by insisting there are many ways of helping people—and by adapting our models to our clients rather than vice versa.

Components of a Common Factors Training Program

An Understanding of Principles of Change

Mastering even *one* model of therapy—let alone several—can be daunting. This task can be made easier by understanding the *principles of change* that pertain across a variety of models (Christensen, Doss, & Atkins, 2005). Beutler et al. (2002) say that principles of change

> identify the conditions, therapist behaviors, and classes of intervention that are associated with change under identified circumstances and for particular kinds of patients. Principles are not theories—they are descriptions of observed relationships. They are more general than techniques and they are more specific than theories. They are the "if ... then" relationships that tell us when to do and what to do, and who to do it to. (p. 3)

In other words, principles are concentrated "truths" of therapeutic change that are characteristic of diverse models and applicable in a wide variety of circumstances. An example of a principle of change in couple and family therapy would be "Couples enjoy greater satisfaction as they free themselves from destructive interactional cycles by slowing down the cycle, standing meta to themselves and their partner, and taking personal responsibility for changing their role in the cycle" (Davis & Piercy, 2007b).

We believe beginning therapists can be taught principles of change as they learn the models within which those principles lie (see Castonguay & Beutler, 2006b, for a thorough discussion of principles of change; Christensen et al., 2005, also provide an informative discussion of principles of change in couple and family therapy). Effective therapists have a solid grasp of principles of change that enables them to adapt to a wide variety of clients and presenting problems. Learning principles of change can help a therapist follow his or her intuition *and* be theory-driven at the same time—two aspects of therapy that are often viewed as being opposite to each other.

An Understanding of Distressed and Healthy Couples

Ask a group of relational therapists "What makes a healthy relationship?" and you'll likely get widely varying opinions with little grounding in data. That is discomforting since we're supposed to be experts on relationships (after all, medical doctors can define "physical health"!). Strangely, since that is what we "treat," many relational therapists are still largely ignorant of the literature on healthy and distressed couples (Gottman & Notarious, 2000). A common factors training program would expose students to the commonalities of healthy and distressed couples. Students could also learn how different models conceptualize these common processes and can be used to intervene to help clients move from distress to a condition of health.

An Understanding of Nonclinical Family Related Research

No model of therapy can address all aspects of the human experience. Therefore it is important for a clinician to be fluent in the literature related to normative human development, gender and diversity issues, spirituality, culture, religion, family studies, communications, relevant sociopolitical issues affecting the family, and so on (Blow et al., 2007).

An Understanding of Broad Common Factors

Students should have a grasp of broad (i.e., those aspects of therapy inherent in the therapy process itself) as well as narrow common factors (i.e., those factors related to the model of therapy, such as common interventions). Therapists should understand how to build, monitor, and maintain the therapeutic alliance, how to engage clients, and how to generate hope and expectancy, among other things.

Self-of-the-Therapist Work

Any training will be of little use if a therapist's work is hindered by unresolved personal issues. In fact, many broad common factors (e.g., establishing a healthy therapeutic alliance) presuppose an emotionally healthy therapist (Timm & Blow, 1999). We believe that ongoing self-of-the-therapist work is an important part of training for both students and educators. We commend programs that strongly encourage students to seek personal therapy during their training, and have arrangements with therapists in the community or through university counseling services that offer reduced fees for students. We also agree with programs that integrate self-of-the-therapist work into courses such as practicum, group therapy, and elsewhere throughout the curriculum.

Practical Examples of Our
Common Factors Training Approach

We have developed an approach to teaching models this way in a master's-level couple therapy course. We are sure there are other ways as well. In our course, students learn approximately one model each week, starting chronologically with the early couple and family therapy models (e.g., Mental Research Institute, Bowen family systems theory, etc.) and ending with today's popular models (e.g., emotionally focused therapy, solution-focused therapy, cognitive-behavioral marital therapy). Having the chronological development of the class follow the chronological development of the field of marital and family therapy enables students to see how each model builds on the strengths of previous models (or at least re-words them!) and attempts to expand on their perceived weaknesses. Each week students are required to turn in an assignment in which they answer the following questions from the perspective of that week's model:

1. Couples have problems because _____?
2. Couples are healthy when _____ (i.e., what do you look for to know when to terminate therapy?).
3. What interventions should you use, and are those interventions aimed at altering affect, cognition, behavior, or something else altogether?
4. What is the therapist's role and the client's role in change?
5. What does this model share in common with other models discussed this semester (in terms of the previous questions and other ways)? What does it add that is unique?
6. What are your likes and dislikes about the model?

Class discussion focuses on the answers to these questions as well as learning the theory and techniques of that model. Furthermore, we discuss how the model could be adapted to various cultures, ethnicities, family forms, and so forth. We also spend several days talking about broad common factors (Davis & Piercy, 2007b) and reviewing the literature related to healthy and distressed couples to see if each model's definitions of "health" and "dysfunction" fit with the larger literature on the subject (Gottman & Notarious, 2000). Though students often complain about the workload, they report feeling more comfortable and competent when using different models than they did prior to undertaking this approach.

Another exercise in this class helps students to learn that models are more similar than different. To achieve this end, students spend time reviewing the literature on healthy and distressed couples. Small groups of students draw on this literature to each pick one to two patterns of healthy or distressed couples. These groups then try to find different models that describe the same patterns of distress and health. Students continue on this path until they have exhausted all of the patterns of health and dysfunction and marital and family therapy models. They also spend time discussing which interventions specific to each model would be used to facilitate movement from dysfunction to health (see Chapter 8 for more on this topic). For example, the Bowenian concept of differentiation (Kerr & Bowen, 1988) generally refers to an individual's ability to distinguish thinking from feeling and, when anxiety is high, to rely on thinking processes rather than being emotionally reactive. People with low differentiation manage their anxiety in relationships by either becoming enmeshed with or distancing themselves from their partner. Similarly, Gottman and Notarious (2000) describe different types of distressed couples. The first is a couple that has a high rate of contingency in their interactions, meaning that one partner's response elicits a similar response from the other partner. In Bowenian terms, they are fused. Another type of distressed couple keeps all of their feelings bottled inside themselves in order to avoid conflict and does not engage in many positive behaviors with each other. In Bowenian terms they are experiencing emotional cutoff.

The literature on healthy and distressed relationships is replete with processes that have been described for a long time by family and couple theories, yet in our experience they are not often treated as two intertwined bodies of literature. We have found that having students integrate them is a nice way to help students know at what points they will likely be starting with a couple and toward what ends they will likely be working. We find that this also helps students to realize that many models are using different language to describe the same couple processes. This can help clinical models seem more similar than different, thus making their integration and flexible use more likely.

Implications for Supervision

Since many of you may not work in training institutions but may supervise therapists as one of your professional roles, we offer some implications for supervisors here. Of course, supervision is often a subcategory of training, so these remarks are also applicable for those who do supervision in a training setting.

Just as a therapist can be a common factors therapist while still being a proponent of a specific model of therapy, you can also supervise from the perspective of a particular model, provided you understand the moderate common factors position on models. Quite frequently, and especially outside of training institutions, supervisors are challenged to work with supervisees who engage in practice using diverse models. We think that having a common-factors-driven paradigm will aid you in working with supervisees from different models since you can go "meta" to these models and recognize their similarities.

We believe supervisors can use the common factors lens in two ways. First, you can ask supervisees the same questions that we suggest in Chapter 12 that therapists ask themselves to monitor their own work from a common factors perspective. (You may wish to turn to Chapter 12, pp. 176–177, for a complete list of these questions. Please also check out Appendix A, where we provide a checklist for supervisors who are using the moderate common factors framework.)

What follows are a few sample questions from the first three of six categories of questions:

1. *Client Characteristics:* "Are my clients engaged and motivated to bring about change? If not, what can I do to match their motivation and stage of readiness for change?"

2. *Therapist Characteristics:* "Am I using a sufficiently high level of activity so as to interrupt dysfunctional patterns and encourage family members to face their cognitive, emotional, and behavioral issues, yet not so much that I am overly controlling or inviting defensiveness?"

3. *The Therapeutic Alliance:* "Am I on the same page as my clients regarding the goals of therapy?"; "Are my tasks credible to my clients?"; "Is our emotional bond strong enough that the clients feel safe?"

Note that these questions are just as applicable to a narrative supervisee as to a solution-focused supervisee or to someone who describes him- or herself as "integrative" or "eclectic." We frequently use these questions as a template for the process of supervision. We believe that they have helped us to approach the process of supervision more systematically and comprehensively, and also that supervisees find the questions helpful and stimulating.

Second, supervisors can modify many of the same questions and apply them to their professional relationship with their supervisees (Walter Lowe, Jr., personal communication, September 2005). For example, as a supervisor you might ask, "Am I on the same page with the supervisee about the goals of supervision?"; "Are my suggestions credible to the supervisee?"; "Have I helped the supervisee to feel hopeful about this case?"; "If the case is painful for the supervisee in some way, does my emotional bond with the supervisee create enough safety to facilitate affective expression?" You can use these common-factors-based questions either internally to monitor your relationship with your supervisee, or you may explicitly choose to ask supervisees some of these questions when you think it is appropriate.

A Climate of Reflective Theoretical Inclusivity

Perhaps the most important component of a common factors training program would be a faculty that fostered a climate of reflective theoretical inclusivity. Students in such an environment would feel less pressure to pick one model and avoid others based on faculty allegiance. It is ironic that, as relationship experts, faculty members and supervisors sometimes refuse to get along with one another solely because they differ on model preferences! In contrast, faculty members in an ideal common factors training program would each be expert in several preferred approaches and would view one another's expertise in different approaches as an asset rather than a source of contention. Faculty members might still engage in lively debate about the efficacy of their preferred models, but this give-and-take would be in the spirit of keeping colleagues and students "on their toes" rather than sowing division. Training programs that offer only one type of training (e.g., postmodern, psychoanalytic, etc.) and ignore or avoid others are incongruent with our common factors approach. The climate created by an inclusive theoretical approach communicates to students the principle that, ironically, relational theorists have struggled with for decades: that by viewing one another's theoretical differences as an opportunity to learn rather than as a threat, we end up being stronger and more well rounded than we would otherwise be.

12

Implications for Clinicians and Researchers

In the first chapter of this book, we laid out an emerging paradigm, common-factors-driven change, that we contrasted with the older model-driven change paradigm. In Chapters 3–11 we spelled out the specifics of this distinction and our primary thesis that common factors are what are primarily responsible for therapeutic change. This chapter will further specify the previously discussed implications of this paradigm shift as well as offer additional implications for clinicians and researchers.

We tried to be clear, especially in Chapter 5 ("A Moderate View of Common Factors") and Chapter 9 ("A Meta-Model of Change in Couple Therapy"), that we are primarily presenting a "meta-model," or way of looking at models from a higher level of abstraction, rather than advocating for another competing model of therapy. Recall from Chapter 1 that these alternate paradigms typically use the same ingredients but view them differently. The common-factors-driven paradigm of change views the same phenomena as the older paradigm—models, clients, therapists, interventions, and the process of change—but sees their interrelations differently. Models are still valuable—even though they are not the primary engine that drives change. For this reason, it will not be necessary for you as a clinician, supervisor, or researcher to make radical changes in what you do in order to follow this emerging paradigm; and we certainly do not want to contribute to the aforementioned tendency in the field to "throw out the baby with the bathwater." The moderate view of common factors (discussed at length in Chapter 5) clearly asserts that common factors work through models and many models are very effective. We have also made it clear that you "gotta have a model." If you are clear about what primarily drives change, you can still hold the common-factors-driven paradigm while calling yourself a proponent of emotionally focused therapy, narrative therapy, functional family therapy, internal family systems therapy, an integrative model, or whatever approach gives your work coherence and structure while offering your clients a credible plan to move them from dysfunction to health. We hope it will be valuable, however, for you to look at your model through the broader lens of the meta-model we have offered here.

General Implications for Clinicians

Practice Professional Modesty

Until and unless there is a lot better evidence than is currently available about the *relative* efficacy of models, making claims for the "superiority" of "my" model is seldom warranted. We hope that this volume will contribute to ending whatever remnants of professional hubris may remain in our field. Just as we argued (in Chapter 11) for inclusivity within therapy training programs, here we call for that spirit in the field at large. We hope that theory-centric squabbling can be replaced by respect, dialogue, and a wider appreciation for the contributions of a variety of approaches, as well as recognition that there are many ways to activate the common factors that are primarily responsible for therapeutic change.

Of course, as "evidence people," we are open to the possibility that future research will show that certain couple and family therapy models offer specific advantages *relative* to other models for certain types of clients and issues—a reasonably well established finding for a few problems within individual therapy (see Chapters 5 and 10). If and when we have this evidence, we should welcome it. We have also indicated that certain *categories* of relational therapy (like present-centered problem-focused ecological models) may be advantageous for some problems (like adolescent conduct disorders) even though the specific models within these general categories have not yet offered evidence of *relative* efficacy. But even if these specific contributions are established, we think it is unlikely they will ever be demonstrated to trump common factors in accounting for favorable outcomes in psychotherapy (see Chapters 5 and 10). So, again, professional modesty about the superiority of specific models is appropriate.

But what if one's practice uses an untested model? We wish that all models would be tested for absolutely efficacy (i.e., offer evidence that they "work" relative to at least some control condition) since some widely practiced models (such as "boot camp" approaches to adolescent conduct disorders) have been shown to be not only non-efficacious but downright harmful (Henggeler, & Sheidow, 2002). However, such findings are rare. We argued in Chapter 10 that few reputable widely practiced contemporary treatments based on sound psychosocial principles are found to be not effective when studied empirically. So, it is quite likely that largely untested models like Bowen therapy, narrative therapy, or internal family systems therapy (if applied in an organized and coherent manner by skilled clinicians) would prove to be just as efficacious as current ESTs. We presented evidence in Chapters 4 and 10 that interpersonal and experiential treatments for depression have proved as potent as the more widely tested cognitive-behavior therapy. Certain models are "assumed" to be superior by virtue of their being tested a lot. If you practice an empirically validated approach, we applaud you; but we also encourage you to be noncommittal or at least modest regarding whether your model is superior to an untested approach. Furthermore, all the evidence we have marshaled in this book leads us confidently to predict that therapists using one of the aforementioned untested models, but maximizing the common factors stressed in this volume, would achieve better results than therapists using previously established ESTs that were deficient in the common factors. Again, the lesson is: be modest about your model.

Choose a Model (or Meta-Model) That You Believe In

While this advice might seem to contradict the preceding guideline, it does not really when interpreted as "for yourself" (as opposed to for everyone). We have mentioned several times in this volume that from a clinical perspective having an "allegiance" to a model may make you more confident and credible and hence enhance the common factor of hope or expectation for change in your clients. We also think there is value to Simon's (2006) argument that using a model that is a good match for your world view may enhance efficacy, provided that it also matches your client's world view, although there is as yet little direct empirical evidence for this claim.

Practice Your Model Flexibly

The primary caveat to this guideline is that you use your preferred model flexibly. The more nonintegrative your model, the more important it is to recognize that narrow models will seldom address effectively the full range of human problems and differences among clients. While a highly integrative model such as Pinsof's (1995) integrative problem-centered model, which incorporates a wide range of existing models, may be applicable to most clients and issues, less integrative approaches will sometimes be a poor match and run the risk of being the proverbial "hammer that turns everything into a nail." The more nonintegrative your model of choice, then, the more likely you will have to reach beyond it to succeed with some clients. This is why we argued in Chapter 11 for the need to be well versed in several models. We also believe it is important to have a well-thought-out rationale about how to integrate these models that is linked to dealing with specific cases.

We have also reviewed the compelling evidence in this book that therapists need to adapt to varying client preferences for directiveness as well as varying client needs for emotional arousal or calmness; and we have reviewed research that some clients respond better to more insight-oriented approaches while others prefer skill-based or symptom-focused methods. Most of Chapter 6 was devoted to showing how some models may work better when clients are at a certain stage of readiness for change (although there is as yet little empirical evidence for matching the particular stage with couple and family therapies) and how important it may be to use different methods to motivate specific clients. We have also been emphatic throughout that therapists must continually adapt to gender, culture, and other diversity issues. Unless your model happens to be highly flexible on these dimensions, then you will have to compensate through your own flexibility.

Get as Much Honest Feedback as You Can

A great contribution of common factors and progress researcher Michael Lambert and colleagues (Harmon, Hawkins, Lambert, Slade, & Whipple, 2005; Lambert, 2005; Lambert et al., 2005) is that therapists do better work when they get honest feedback about how they are doing. This conclusion seems to hold true for whatever models the therapists are employing, which also supports the common factors view of change since the improvement effects cut across all models. The very process of getting the feedback seems to make therapists more conscious of doing good work and more determined to achieve favorable results.

While it would be advantageous for all therapists to use well-validated assessment instruments regularly (though some measures of outcome and of the therapeutic alliance are very short-term and practical; see Appendix 5 of Duncan & Miller, 2000) realistically this need is unlikely to be met in nonmandated settings. However, therapists should not rely on spontaneous informal client feedback since it tends to be favorably biased and seldom calls for needed change. Even if using an assessment instrument (and perhaps more importantly when therapists ask for feedback orally), they should communicate to their clients a message like:

> "I would appreciate some honest feedback from you. Often clients want to please their therapists by saying nice things, but this is not very helpful when there are issues about therapy that might call for some changes. I would value learning what is *not* helpful in our work as well as what is helpful. So, I would be grateful if you would be willing to give me honest and specific feedback about our work together and our relationship."

Therapists should also ask clients regularly what has been "pivotal" (Helmeke & Sprenkle, 2000) in therapy since, as we have already noted several times, client perceptions about what has been significant in therapy are often dramatically different from our own.

In addition to the data that honest feedback provides the typical therapist, there is also some evidence that the very best therapists— the true superstars of the profession—are much more attuned to client feedback than average or even superior therapists. They are much more conscientious about getting feedback about how the client feels about them and their work (and they don't, like so many therapists, just *say* that they do); more importantly, they work harder at using this feedback to actually *improve* their performance (Miller, Hubble, & Duncan, 2007).

Specific Implications for Clinicians

For a specific example of how our common factors approach has affected how we do couple therapy, see Chapter 9. What follows are some additional specific things you can do as a therapist who views your work through a common factors lens. Most of the guidelines will be presented as a series of questions that you can ask yourself to monitor your work and then take appropriate action.

Capitalize on the Common Factors Unique to Relationship Therapy

Since most of the readers of this book are likely to be couple and family therapists, we hope that you will take advantage of the four unique common factors that we described in Chapter 3: (1) conceptualizing difficulties in relational terms, (2) disrupting dysfunctional relational patterns, (3) expanding the direct treatment system, and (4) expanding the therapeutic alliance. These four common factors are essential to the development of relationship therapy and every effective couple and family therapy approach capitalizes on them. Indeed, without them relationship therapy would not exist.

Since becoming more common-factors-driven in our own clinical work as relational therapists, based on these four unique factors we have begun asking ourselves a simple series of questions with each case that we have encountered. An integral part of looking at problems relationally is understanding the dysfunctional cycles in which the problems are embedded, and merely asking the question "What are the dysfunctional cycles that are maintaining this problem, and how can I facilitate the clients' disrupting them?" is likely to advance your work. Capitalizing on expanding the direct treatment system while also keeping in mind the important characters in the indirect system who are not present but who are crucial to the "problem maintenance structure" (Pinsof, 1995) is also a good idea. "Who needs to be included in this therapy to capitalize on the interactional view?" Finally, paying attention to the unique aspects of the therapeutic alliance when multiple persons are involved, like keeping it balanced and avoiding "split" alliances, should pay rich dividends. "What is my alliance like with the various family members and subsystems, and are my alliances balanced or are they split?"

Capitalize on the Broad as Well as the Narrow View of Common Factors

When most people think of common factors, what comes to mind is either the narrow view (mechanisms of change that are common to all models, although the language and techniques look different on the surface—described in detail in Chapter 8) or the therapeutic relationship or alliance (the subject of Chapter 7). These are only two aspects of a six-part broader view of common factors that we outlined in Chapter 4.

Here, again, we are asking ourselves and our supervisees the questions that follow that capitalize on the broad view of the common factors paradigm. (Recall that we have emphasized that the categories below are not distinct but interact with one another.) We stress again that this is a meta-framework and that you can ask these questions regardless of your preferred model(s) for doing psychotherapy.

1. *Client Characteristics:* "Are my clients engaged and motivated to bring about change? If not, what can I do to match their motivation and stage of readiness for change?" "Is my conceptualization of the nature of their problem too much of a stretch for them? If they don't 'buy it,' how do I adapt to them?"; "Do I regularly assess what they think is not helpful as well as helpful about the therapy?" (See Chapters 4 and 6.)

2. *Therapist Characteristics:* "Am I using a sufficiently high level of activity so as to interrupt dysfunctional patterns and provide sufficient structure to encourage family members to face their cognitive, emotional, and behavioral issues, yet not so much that I am appearing overly controlling or inviting defensiveness?"; "Am I keeping the level of emotional arousal in the session moderate (neither too high nor too low)?"; "Am I choosing interventions that are a good match for the learning style of these clients (e.g., insight-oriented vs. skill-building or symptom-focused)?" (See Chapter 4.)

3. *The Therapeutic Alliance:* "Am I on the same page as my clients regarding the goals of therapy?"; "Are my tasks credible to my clients?"; "Is our emotional bond strong enough that the clients feel safe?" (See Chapter 7.)

4. *Hope or Expectancy:* "My clients likely came to therapy demoralized—what have I done to remoralize them?"; "Am I conveying a sense of hope?"; "Do they 'buy' my conceptualization of their problems and the way out of them?" (See Chapter 4.)

5. *Interventions That Cut across Various Models (the narrow view of common factors):* "What have I done to help my clients change the 'viewing' (cognitive change) of their problems?"; "What have I done to help my clients change the 'doing' (behavior change) of their problem?"; "What have I done to facilitate affective expression, or regulation, or attachment?" (affective change). (See Chapter 8.) Regardless of the specific

methods you may use to interrupt dysfunctional cycles, you might ask: "Have I helped family members to 'slow down' the process?"; "Have I helped family members to stand meta (or develop a self-observing stance) to their own process?"; "Have I encouraged family members to take personal responsibility for their own contributions to the dysfunctional cycle?" (See Chapter 9.)

6. *Other Mediating and Moderating Variables (Allegiance and Organization/Coherence):* "Do I have a sincere belief in my approach that both enables me to 'sell' my view of the problem and its remediation and also seems credible to my clients?"; "Is my approach organized and coherent enough to give me confidence that I know what I am doing, and do I inspire this same confidence in my clients?" (See Chapter 4.)

General Implications for Researchers

Embed Common Factors Research into Individual Studies

Throughout this volume we have stressed that there is a strong research base for the general thesis that common factors are what primarily drive therapeutic change. However, most of this evidence comes from meta-analysis—conclusions based on aggregate data from a large number of studies, most of which were not, as individual investigations, specifically studying common factors. With the exception of research on the therapeutic alliance, there are not many individual studies that deliberately focus on the major common factors described in this book.

So, our first recommendation is that researchers study the major common factors intentionally in individual investigations. Practically speaking, however, in the short run researchers may need to embed common factors research into research designs on topics that are more fundable. Like it or not, NIH funding is currently focused on treatments related to DSM diagnoses. It is unlikely in the current environment that studies primarily focused on common factors will be funded, at least by NIH. However, as we noted in Chapters 5 and 10, there is nothing inherent in clinical trials methods for investigating treatments of DSM diagnosable problems that would prevent researchers from studying some common factors like client factors, differential therapist efficacy, and so forth. Of course, as noted in Chapter 10, some common factors cannot be experimentally manipulated in ethical research. Blow and associates (2007) offer several additional specific suggestions for embedding research on some common factors variables into clinical trials research.

Continue Support for Randomized Clinical Trials and Empirically Supported Psychotherapies, But with Caveats

We emphasized in Chapters 5 and 10 that there is value in randomized clinical trials. The moderate common factors position stresses that models still have a responsibility to establish "absolute" efficacy even when "relative" efficacy is not known or proven. Furthermore, the only way that couple and family therapies will establish credibility with such external audiences as the scientific community, governments, and third-party payers, is by using so-called gold-standard methods for establishing efficacy and effectiveness. We also believe, for the pragmatic reason mentioned in the preceding paragraph, that clinical trials research will continue to be funded and researchers can embed common factors research into these designs. Meta-analyses based on clinical trials will also continue to provide valuable data regarding the common factors versus specific factors debate. Furthermore, we emphasized in Chapter 10 that ESTs are the treatment of choice for a limited number of difficult problems where highly specialized treatments are needed.

So, there is no need to take the more radical position that some common factors scholars have taken that clinical trials research and the continued designation of new ESTs should be abandoned. However, we do believe that there should be much greater awareness of the shortcomings of these approaches and their limited value—at least as currently practiced (see Chapter 10 for more details). We are encouraged that highly respected scholars who are not calling for the demise of these methods are writing serious critiques of these approaches in prestigious journals (Westen et al., 2004).

Change the Culture of Research in the Long Run

In Chapter 1 we argued that the existing research establishment predominantly supports the model-driven change paradigm. This paradigm is based on the medical model, which assumes that diagnoses typically lead to clear treatments and that, analogously, psychotherapy research is like "drug research without the drugs." The treatment model is what is important, and such a contextual factor as who delivers the treatment is considered relatively unimportant. Without repeating all of the arguments we made in Chapters 1, 5, and 10, suffice it to say here that there are far more important client variables than the client's diagnosis when it comes to impacting outcomes, that therapist variables are hugely important, and that other "common factors" frequently trump the choice of treatment in determining outcomes.

So as long as the researcher *zeitgeist* continues to emphasize the role of treatments at the cost of ignoring these other variables, then we say that this situation cries out for changing the culture of research! We think that in the long run the field and society in general are better served by research that shows how all legitimate treatments can be made more effective as well as by research that gives us a better understanding of how effective treatments really work.

We also think it is unfortunate that it is so difficult to get research funding for most of the typical problems in living that consume our professional time as relationship therapists. For example, getting federal funding for couple therapy research (marital discord) unrelated to a specific DSM diagnosis is becoming very difficult (Andrew Christensen, personal communication, March 20, 2007).

Finally, while honoring the role of randomized clinical trials (as above), we think the culture of research should place more value on progress research (Pinsof & Wynne, 2000) that shows how client outcome and alliance change in therapy on a session-by-session basis and that incorporates the use of feedback to therapists that impacts "their next move." We also believe that qualitative research has a valuable place in the researcher's armamentarium and has great promise for casting light on the key question of what is responsible for therapeutic change (see Davis & Piercy, 2007a, 2007b). Process or observational and outcome research that focuses on common processes across effective therapies also holds promise for shedding light on the *why* and *how* of effective therapy, regardless of the model being employed. Moreover, making the links between existing research outlining common aspects of healthy and dysfunctional couples and couple therapy models more explicit could greatly further our understanding of how to use our therapy models to help people change.

None of these changes in the culture of research will be easy or accomplished quickly. We hope that the excellent work of the scholars we have cited in this book, as well as this volume itself, will help to legitimize these changes. If you believe in these ideas, we hope you will publicize and support them.

Specific Implications for Researchers

What follows are some representative, but by no means exhaustive, research questions that we hope investigators will tackle in the years ahead, based on the categories of common factors set forth in this volume. For more ideas see the research reviews in Chapters 4, 7, and 10. Once again, all of these questions apply to any couple and family therapy model, and we also recognize that there are no clear distinctions among the following categories.

1. *Client Characteristics:* "How, in relationship therapy, is the outcome impacted by the client's readiness to change and level of motivation or engagement in therapy?"; "What is the impact of client characteristics like perseverance, willingness to do homework, inner strength, and so on?" (See Chapter 6.)

2. *Therapist Characteristics:* "Independent of the model employed, what (other than the ability to form strong alliances and to be flexible/adaptable) distinguishes superior from average relationship therapists?" (See Chapter 4.) "Are the results achieved by relationship therapists positively impacted by getting session-by-session client feedback (as is the case for the results achieved by individual therapists)?"

3. *The Therapeutic Alliance:* "How does therapist sensitivity to the multiple alliances in couple and family therapy impact outcome?"; "How is the 'tear-and-repair' mechanism that improves the alliance in individual therapy impacted by 'split' alliances in relationship therapy?" (See Chapter 7.)

4. *Hope or Expectancy:* "How specifically can therapists 'remoralize' demoralized couples and families?"; "What is the longitudinal course of hope in relationship therapy? For example, in successful therapy, is hope typically established early and maintained?" (See Chapter 4.)

5. *Interventions That Cut across Various Models (the Narrow View of Common Factors):* "Do all couple and family therapies use behavioral, cognitive, and affective mechanisms to interrupt dysfunctional cycles?" (See Chapter 8.) "When cycles are interrupted, do family members perceive that they have 'slowed down the process,' 'stood meta to their process,' and 'assumed personal responsibility'?" (See Chapter 9.)

6. *Other Mediating and Moderating Variables (Allegiance and*

Organization/Coherence): "How does the effect size of 'allegiance' in relationship therapy compare with the effect size of 'treatment' variables?"; "How can 'organization/coherence' be operationalized, and what is its relationship to outcomes in relationship therapy?" (See Chapter 4.)

Whether or not you have completed the same paradigm shift that we have, we hope you are now looking at your work through a different lens and asking new questions. If our thesis is correct, the emerging paradigm will have significant implications not only for therapists and how they view their work but also for trainers, supervisors, and researchers. We also think this approach has significant implications for the field in general and over time may well affect how external audiences like funding agencies and third-party payers come to view couple and family therapy and psychotherapy more broadly.

Is this emerging paradigm complete? Hardly! Although we think there is compelling evidence for the general thesis that common factors are what primarily drive therapeutic change, our knowledge of the specifics of this process is informed only by incipient research and development. Even at the theoretical level, we acknowledge that the meta-model that we describe in Chapter 9 was developed for couple therapy, and aspects of it may not apply to family therapy. The research evidence for the application of many of the specific dimensions of common factors to relationship therapy is still in its infancy. This is true, however, even for empirically supported relationship therapies like emotionally focused therapy. We know that that therapy works, but we are much less confident about the contributions of specific ingredients. For common factors as well as the models that activate and use them, theory and practice will probably always be well ahead of the evidence that backs them.

These limitations notwithstanding, we think that the evidence for common factors is compelling enough that we hope theoreticians will continue to refine these ideas, that clinicians will try them out, and that researchers will test them. We have offered many specific suggestions in this final chapter. We have always believed that the field will advance through the synergy of theory, research, and practice. We hope that this volume contributes to all three of these domains and enriches your own work.

We find it ironic that, as relationship experts, there are some of us who cannot get along with one another based on something the data show is relatively inconsequential—model preference. Although such a stance is understandable in an evidence-deficient emerging profession that is still defining itself in relationship to other fields, we believe that this developmental phase of couple and family therapy is now quickly receding into the past. The field of relational therapy has matured, and it is an accepted and empirically supported discipline for working with a wide array of mental health problems. We believe that the time has come to reflect the field's maturity in our relationships with one another by focusing on what unites us. By actively fostering inclusivity as it relates to theories, couple and family therapists will be practicing what they preach about the interconnectedness of social systems. If what relational therapists preach has any merit—and we are confident that it does—then our inclusive common factors approach can only bring greater unity to the field in the process of also benefiting couples and families immensely.

Appendix A

Moderate Common Factors Supervision Checklist

SUPERVISEE GOALS

Below are several questions and goals inspired by a moderate common factors framework. List the degree to which you have attained this goal, both at the beginning and the end of the semester.

Client Characteristics

1. Are my style and interventions matched with the client's level of motivation? If not, what can I do to match their motivation and stage of readiness for change?

Beginning: 1   2   3   4   5   6   7   8   9   10
   Not proficient   *Proficient*

End: 1   2   3   4   5   6   7   8   9   10
   Not proficient   *Proficient*

Comments:

2. Is my conceptualization of the nature of their problem too much of a stretch for them?

Beginning: 1   2   3   4   5   6   7   8   9   10
    Not proficient   *Proficient*

End: 1   2   3   4   5   6   7   8   9   10
    Not proficient   *Proficient*

Comments:

3. If my clients don't "buy" my conceptualization, am I adapting it to them? What specifically am I doing to accomplish this?

Beginning: 1   2   3   4   5   6   7   8   9   10
    Not proficient   *Proficient*

End: 1   2   3   4   5   6   7   8   9   10
    Not proficient   *Proficient*

Comments:

4. Do I regularly assess what my clients think is not helpful as well as helpful about the therapy?

Beginning: 1   2   3   4   5   6   7   8   9   10
    Not proficient   *Proficient*

End: 1   2   3   4   5   6   7   8   9   10
    Not proficient   *Proficient*

Comments:

Therapist Characteristics

1. Am I using a sufficiently high level of activity and structure so as to interrupt dysfunctional patterns and encourage family members to face their

cognitive, emotional, and behavioral issues, yet not so much that I am overly controlling or inviting defensiveness?

Beginning: 1   2   3   4   5   6   7   8   9   10
    Not proficient   *Proficient*

End: 1   2   3   4   5   6   7   8   9   10
    Not proficient   *Proficient*

Comments:

2. Am I keeping the level of emotional arousal in the session moderate (neither too high nor too low)?

Beginning: 1   2   3   4   5   6   7   8   9   10
    Not proficient   *Proficient*

End: 1   2   3   4   5   6   7   8   9   10
    Not proficient   *Proficient*

Comments:

3. Am I choosing interventions that are a good match for the learning style of these clients (e.g., insight-oriented vs. skill-building/symptom-focused)?

Beginning: 1   2   3   4   5   6   7   8   9   10
    Not proficient   *Proficient*

End: 1   2   3   4   5   6   7   8   9   10
    Not proficient   *Proficient*

Comments:

The Therapeutic Alliance

1. Am I on the same page as my clients regarding the goals of therapy?

Beginning: 1   2   3   4   5   6   7   8   9   10
     Not proficient   *Proficient*

End: 1   2   3   4   5   6   7   8   9   10
     Not proficient   *Proficient*

Comments:

2. Are my tasks credible to my clients?

Beginning: 1   2   3   4   5   6   7   8   9   10
     Not proficient   *Proficient*

End: 1   2   3   4   5   6   7   8   9   10
     Not proficient   *Proficient*

Comments:

3. Is our emotional bond strong enough that the clients feel safe?

Beginning: 1   2   3   4   5   6   7   8   9   10
     Not proficient   *Proficient*

End: 1   2   3   4   5   6   7   8   9   10
     Not proficient   *Proficient*

Comments:

Hope or Expectancy

1. If my clients came to therapy demoralized, am I taking specific steps to remoralize them?

Beginning: 1   2   3   4   5   6   7   8   9   10
     Not proficient   *Proficient*

End: 1   2   3   4   5   6   7   8   9   10
     Not proficient   *Proficient*

Comments:

2. Am I conveying a sense of hope?

Beginning: 1   2   3   4   5   6   7   8   9   10
     Not proficient   *Proficient*

End: 1   2   3   4   5   6   7   8   9   10
     Not proficient   *Proficient*

Comments:

3. Do they believe that the treatment plan provides a credible way out of their problems?

Beginning: 1   2   3   4   5   6   7   8   9   10
     Not proficient   *Proficient*

End: 1   2   3   4   5   6   7   8   9   10
     Not proficient   *Proficient*

Comments:

Interventions That Cut across Various Models

1. If applicable, am I helping my clients change the "viewing" (cognitive change) of their problems?

Beginning: 1   2   3   4   5   6   7   8   9   10
    Not proficient   Proficient

End: 1   2   3   4   5   6   7   8   9   10
    Not proficient   Proficient

Comments:

2. If applicable, what am I doing to help my clients change the "doing" (behavior change) of their problems?

Beginning: 1   2   3   4   5   6   7   8   9   10
    Not proficient   Proficient

End: 1   2   3   4   5   6   7   8   9   10
    Not proficient   Proficient

Comments:

3. If applicable, am I facilitating healthy affective expression, regulation, or attachment (affective change)?

Beginning: 1   2   3   4   5   6   7   8   9   10
    Not proficient   Proficient

End: 1   2   3   4   5   6   7   8   9   10
    Not proficient   Proficient

Comments:

4. Am I helping family members "slow down" their process?

Beginning: 1   2   3   4   5   6   7   8   9   10
    Not proficient   *Proficient*

End: 1   2   3   4   5   6   7   8   9   10
    Not proficient   *Proficient*

Comments:

5. Am I helping family members to stand outside of ("go meta") their own process?

Beginning: 1   2   3   4   5   6   7   8   9   10
    Not proficient   *Proficient*

End: 1   2   3   4   5   6   7   8   9   10
    Not proficient   *Proficient*

Comments:

6. Am I encouraging family members to take personal responsibility for their own contributions to the dysfunctional cycle?

Beginning: 1   2   3   4   5   6   7   8   9   10
    Not proficient   *Proficient*

End: 1   2   3   4   5   6   7   8   9   10
    Not proficient   *Proficient*

Comments:

Other Variables

1. Do I have a sincere belief in my approach that both enables me to "sell" my view of the problem and its remediation, and also seems credible to my clients?

Beginning: 1   2   3   4   5   6   7   8   9   10
    Not proficient   *Proficient*

End: 1   2   3   4   5   6   7   8   9   10
    Not proficient   *Proficient*

Comments:

2. Is my approach organized and coherent enough to give me confidence that I know what I am doing, and inspire this same confidence in my clients?

Beginning: 1   2   3   4   5   6   7   8   9   10
    Not proficient   *Proficient*

End: 1   2   3   4   5   6   7   8   9   10
    Not proficient   *Proficient*

Comments:

Case-Specific Questions and Goals

1. Question/Goal:

Beginning: 1   2   3   4   5   6   7   8   9   10
    Not proficient   *Proficient*

End: 1   2   3   4   5   6   7   8   9   10
    Not proficient   *Proficient*

Comments:

2. Question/Goal:

Beginning: 1   2   3   4   5   6   7   8   9   10
        Not proficient   *Proficient*

End: 1   2   3   4   5   6   7   8   9   10
        Not proficient   *Proficient*

Comments:

3. Question/Goal:

Beginning: 1   2   3   4   5   6   7   8   9   10
        Not proficient   *Proficient*

End: 1   2   3   4   5   6   7   8   9   10
        Not proficient   *Proficient*

Comments:

General Case Comments

Supervisor Comments

Supervisor _____ Date _____

Therapist _____ Date _____

Appendix B

Instruments from Other Authors Related to Common Factors

The Integrative Psychotherapy Alliance Scales developed by Pinsof and colleagues and the Session Rating Scales developed by Miller, Duncan, and colleagues are rating scales for assessing alliance and in-session therapeutic processes that are simple and easy to administer and to score. We reproduce the
short form of the Integrative Psychotherapy Alliance Scales, the most recent
versions of these scales, and the various versions of the Session Rating Scales
developed for adults and children of different ages. These scales are described
in the references below. Permission to utilize these scales should be obtained
from the authors of the scales before reproducing them.

References

Pinsof, W. M., Zinbarg, R., & Knobloch-Fedders, L. M. (2008). Factorial
and construct validity of the revised short form integrative psychotherapy alliance scales for family, couple, and individual therapy. *Family
Process, 47,* 281–301.
Duncan, B. L., Miller, S., & Sparks, J. (2004). *The heroic client: A revolutionary way to improve effectiveness through client-centered, outcome-
informed therapy* (rev. ed.). San Francisco: Jossey-Bass.
www.talkingcure.com. Session Rating Scales. Session Rating Scale (SRS
V.3.0)

Integrative Psychotherapy Alliance Scales—Revised—Short Form

STIC INTERSESSION | Integrative Psychotherapy Alliance Scales-R-SF (Individual, Couple, Family) from STIC® Intersession 2005. The Family Institute. All rights reserved. | PAGE 6

QUESTIONS ABOUT YOUR THERAPY

The following questions refer to your feelings and thoughts about your therapist and your therapy right *now*. Please rate how much you agree or disagree with each statement *now*. Respond to the Individual Therapy questions if you are in individual therapy (most sessions involve just you); respond to the Couples Therapy questions if you are in couples therapy (most sessions involve you and your partner); or respond to the Family Therapy questions if you are in family therapy (most sessions involve you and your family). *Only fill out one of the three groups of questions*.

Completely Disagree
Strongly Disagree
Disagree
Neutral
Agree
Strongly Agree
Completely Agree

INDIVIDUAL THERAPY (most sessions involve just you)

1. Some of the people who are important to me would *not* be pleased with what I am doing in this therapy.
2. The therapist does *not* understand me.
3. Some of the people who are important to me would *not* agree with the therapist about the goals of this therapy.
4. The therapist and I are *not* in agreement about the goals for this therapy.

5. Some of the people who are important to me and I do *not* feel the same way about what I want to get out of this therapy.
6. The people who are important to me would understand my goals in this therapy.
7. Some of the people who are important to me would *not* be accepting of my involvement in this therapy.
8. I do *not* care about the therapist as a person.

9. I do *not* feel accepted by the therapist.
10. Some of the people who are important to me would *not* trust that this therapy is good for my relationships with them.
11. The people who are important to me would approve of the way my therapy is being conducted.
12. The people who are important to me would feel accepted by the therapist.

13. The therapist does *not* agree with the goals I have for my important relationships.
14. The therapist does *not* appreciate how important some of my relationships are to me.
15. The therapist is helping me with my important relationships.
16. I am satisfied with this therapy.

COUPLES THERAPY (most sessions involve you and your partner)

1. The therapist cares about me as a person.
2. The therapist understands my goals in this therapy.
3. The therapist and I are in agreement about the way the therapy is being conducted.
4. The therapist does *not* understand the relationship between my partner and myself.

(continued)

Rating scale (for all items): Completely Agree · Strongly Agree · Agree · Neutral · Disagree · Strongly Disagree · Completely Disagree

COUPLES THERAPY (continued)

5. The therapist cares about the relationship between my partner and myself.
6. The therapist does *not* understand the goals that my partner and I have for ourselves as a couple in this therapy.
7. My partner feels accepted by the therapist.
8. My partner and the therapist are in agreement about the way the therapy is being conducted.
9. The therapist understands my partner's goals for this therapy.
10. My partner and I do *not* accept each other in this therapy.
11. My partner and I are in agreement about our goals for this therapy.
12. My partner and I are *not* pleased with the things that each of us does in this therapy.
13. I am satisfied with this therapy.

FAMILY THERAPY (most sessions involve you and your family)

1. The therapist does *not* understand me.
2. The therapist understands my goals in therapy.
3. I trust the therapist.
4. The therapist does *not* understand my family's goals for this therapy.
5. The therapist lacks the skills and ability to help my family.
6. The therapist cares about my family.
7. The therapist has the skills and ability to help all the other members of my family.
8. The therapist understands the goals that all the other members of my family have for this therapy.
9. The therapist does *not* care personally about some of the other members of my family.
10. Some of the other members of my family and I do *not* feel the same way about what we want to get out of this therapy.
11. Some of the other members of my family and I are *not* pleased with the things that each of us is doing in this therapy.
12. Some of the other members of my family and I do *not* feel safe with each other in this therapy.
13. I am satisfied with this therapy.

(Side tab: QUESTIONS ABOUT YOUR THERAPY)

Session Rating Scale (SRS V.3.0)

Name: _____ Age (Yrs.): _____
ID# _____ Sex: M / F
Session # _____ Date: _____

Please rate today's session by placing a mark on the line nearest to the description that best fits your experience.

Relationship

I did not feel heard, understood, and respected.
|----Examination Copy Only----|
I felt heard, understood, and respected.

Goals and Topics

We did *not* work on or talk about what I wanted to work on and talk about.
|----Examination Copy Only----|
We worked on and talked about what I wanted to work on and talk about.

Approach or Method

The therapist's approach is not a good fit for me.
|----Examination Copy Only----|
The therapist's approach is a good fit for me.

Overall

There was something missing in the session today.
|----Examination Copy Only----|
Overall, today's session was right for me.

Institute for the Study of Therapeutic Change

www.talkingcure.com

Child Session Rating Scale (CSRS)

Name: _____ Age (Yrs.): _____
Sex: M / F
Session # _____ Date: _____

How was our time together today? Please put a mark on the lines below to let us know how you feel.

Listening

Did not always
listen to me.
|---Examination Copy Only---|
Listened to me.

How Important

What we did and
talked about was
not really that
important to me.
|---Examination Copy Only---|
What we did and
talked about
were important
to me.

What We Did

I did not like
what we did
today.
|---Examination Copy Only---|
I liked what
we did today.

Overall

I wish we could do
something
different.
|---Examination Copy Only---|
I hope we do
the same kinds
of things
next time.

Institute for the Study of Therapeutic Change

www.talkingcure.com

Young Child Session Rating Scale (YCSRS)

Name:_____ Age (Yrs.):_____
Sex: M / F
Session #_____ Date:_____

Choose one of the faces that shows how it was for you to be here today. Or, you can
draw one below that is just right for you.

Institute for the Study of Therapeutic Change

www.talkingcure.com

References

Ackerman, N. W. (1970). *Family therapy in transition*. Oxford, England: Little, Brown.

Adler, A. (1951). *The practice and theory of individual psychology* (2nd ed., rev.). Oxford, England: Humanities Press. (Original work published 1924)

Anderson, C. M., Hogarty, G. E., & Reiss, D. J. (1980). Family treatment of adult schizophrenic patients: A psycho-educational approach. *Schizophrenia Bulletin, 6*(3), 490–505.

Annunziata, D., Hogue, A., Faw, L., & Liddle, H. A. (2006). Family functioning and school success in at-risk, inner-city adolescents. *Journal of Youth and Adolescence, 35*(1), 105–113.

Asay, T. P., & Lambert, M. J. (1999). The empirical case for the common factors in therapy. In M. A. Hubble, B. L. Duncan, & S. D. Miller (Eds.), *The heart and soul of change: What works in therapy* (pp. 23–55). Washington, DC: American Psychological Association.

Barlow, D. H., Allen, L. B., & Basden, S. L. (2007). Psychological treatments for panic disorders, phobias, and generalized anxiety disorder. In P. E. Nathan & J. M. Gorman (Eds.), *A guide to treatments that work* (3rd ed., pp. 351–394). New York: Oxford University Press.

Barlow, D. H., Pincus, D. B., Heinrichs, N., & Choate, M. L. (2003). Anxiety disorders. In G. Stricker & T. A. Widiger (Eds.), *Handbook of psychology: Clinical psychology* (pp. 119–147). New York: Wiley.

Barton, C., & Alexander, J. F. (1977). Therapists' skills as determinants of effective systems-behavioral family therapy. *American Journal of Family Therapy, 5*(2), 11–19.

Bateson, G. (1972). *Steps to an ecology of mind: Collected essays in anthropology, psychiatry, evolution, and epistemology*. Northvale, NJ: Jason Aronson.

Beck, A. T., & Weishaar, M. E. (1989). Cognitive therapy. In A. Freeman, K.

M. Simon, L. E. Beutler, & H. Arkowitz (Eds.), *Comprehensive hand-book of cognitive therapy* (pp. 21–36). New York: Plenum Press.

Beutler, L. E., Bongar, B., & Shurkin, J. N. (1998). *A consumer's guide to psychotherapy*. New York: Oxford University Press.

Beutler, L. E., Consoli, A. J., & Lane, J. (2005). Systemic treatment selection and prescriptive psychotherapy. In J. C. Norcross & M. R. Goldfried (Eds.), *Handbook of psychotherapy integration* (2nd ed., pp. 121–143). New York: Oxford University Press.

Beutler, L. E., Harwood, T. M., Alimohamed, S., & Malik, M. (2002). Functional impairment and coping style. In J. Norcross (Ed.), *Psychotherapy relationships that work: Therapist contributions and responsiveness to patient needs* (pp. 145–170). New York: Oxford University Press.

Beutler, L. E., Malik, M. L., & Alimohamed, S. (2004). Therapist variables. In M. J. Lambert (Ed.), *Bergin and Garfield's handbook of psychotherapy and behavior change* (pp. 227–306). New York: Wiley.

Bischoff, R. J., & Sprenkle, D. H. (1993). Dropping out of marriage and family therapy: A critical view of research. *Family Process, 32,* 353–375.

Blatt, S. J., Sanislow, C. A., Zuroff, D. C., & Pilkonis, P. A. (1996). Characteristics of effective therapists: Further analyses of data from the National Institute of Mental Health treatment of depression collaborative research program. *Journal of Consulting and Clinical Psychology, 64,* 1276–1284.

Blow, A. J., Davis, S. D., & Sprenkle, D. H. (in press). Therapist worldview: A fruitless dialogue without more evidence. *Journal of Marital and Family Therapy.*

Blow, A. J., Sprenkle, D. H., & Davis, S. D. (2007). Is who delivers the treatment more important than the treatment itself?: The role of the therapist in common factors. *Journal of Marital and Family Therapy, 33,* 298–317.

Boszormenyi-Nagy, I., & Spark, G. M. (1973). *Invisible loyalties: Reciprocity in intergenerational family therapy*. Oxford, England: Harper & Row.

Bowen, M. (1960). A family concept of schizophrenia. In D. Jackson (Ed.), *The etiology of schizophrenia* (pp. 346–372). Oxford, England: Basic Books.

Bowen, M. (1972). Family therapy and family group therapy. In H. I. Kaplan & B. J. Sadock (Eds.), *Group treatment of mental illness* (pp. 384–421). New York: Dutton.

Bowen, M. (1974). Alcoholism as viewed through family systems theory and family psychotherapy. *Annals of the New York Academy of Sciences, 233,* 115–122.

Bowen, M. (1978). *Family therapy in clinical practice*. New York: Jason Aronson.

Bowlby, J. (1988). *A secure base*. New York: Basic Books.

Boyd-Franklin, N. (2003). *Black families in therapy: Understanding the African American experience* (2nd ed.). New York: Guilford Press.

Breunlin, D. C., & Mac Kune-Karrer, B. (2002). Metaframeworks. In F. W. Kaslow (Ed.), *Comprehensive handbook of psychotherapy: Vol. 4. Integrative/eclectic* (pp. 367–385). New York: Wiley.

Breunlin, D. C., Schwartz, R. C., & Mac Kune-Karrer, B. (1997). *Metaframeworks: Transcending the models of family therapy* (rev., & updated). San Francisco: Jossey-Bass.

Butler, M. H., & Bird, M. H. (2000). Narrative and interactional process for preventing harmful struggle in therapy: An integrative model. *Journal of Marital and Family Therapy, 26,* 123–142.

Castonguay, L. G., & Beutler, L. E. (2006a). Principles of therapeutic change: A task force on participants, relationships, and technique factors. *Journal of Clinical Psychology, 62*(6), 631–638.

Castonguay, L. G., & Beutler, L. E. (2006b). *Principles of therapeutic change that work.* New York: Oxford University Press.

Chamberlain, P. (2003). Multidimensional treatment foster care program components and principles of practice. In P. Chamberlain (Ed.), *Treating chronic juvenile offenders: Advances made through the Oregon multidimensional treatment foster care model law and public policy* (pp. 69–93). Washington, DC: American Psychological Association.

Chamberlain, P., & Smith, D. K. (2005). Multidimensional treatment foster care: A community solution for boys and girls referred from juvenile justice. In E. D. Hibbs & P. S. Jensen (Eds.), *Psychosocial treatments for child and adolescent disorders: Empirically based strategies for clinical practice* (2nd ed., pp. 557–573). Washington, DC: American Psychological Association.

Chambless, D. L. (1999). Empirically validated treatments—what now? *Applied and Preventive Psychology, 8*(4), 281–284.

Chambless, D. L. (2002). Beware the dodo bird: The dangers of overgeneralization. *Clinical Psychology: Science and Practice, 9*(1), 13–16.

Chambless, D. L., & Hollon, S. D. (1998). Defining empirically supported therapies. *Journal of Consulting and Clinical Psychology, 66,* 7–18.

Chambless, D. L., & Ollendick, T. H. (2001). Empirically supported psychological interventions: Controversies and evidence. *Annual Review of Psychology, 52,* 685–716.

Christensen, A., Atkins, D. C., Berns, S., Wheeler, J., Baucom, D. H., & Simpson, L. E. (2004). Traditional versus integrative behavioral couple therapy for significantly and chronically distressed married couples. *Journal of Consulting and Clinical Psychology, 72*(2), 176–191.

Christensen, A., Doss, B. D., & Atkins, D. C. (2005). A science of couple therapy: For what should we seek empirical support? In W. M. Pinsof & J. L. Lebow (Eds.), *Family psychology: The art of the science* (pp. 43–63). New York: Oxford University Press.

Clarkin, J. F., & Levy, K. N. (2004). Research on client variables in psychotherapy. In M. J. Lambert (Ed.), *Bergin and Garfield's handbook of psychotherapy and behavior change* (pp. 194–226). New York: Wiley.

Combs, G., & Freidman, J. (1998). Tellings and retellings. *Journal of Marital and Family Therapy, 24*(4), 405–408.

Crane, R. D., Griffin, W., & Hill, R. D. (1986). Influence of therapist skills on client perceptions of marriage and family therapy outcome: Implications for supervision. *Journal of Marital and Family Therapy, 12,* 91–96.

Craske, M. G., & Barlow, D. H. (2001). Panic disorder and agoraphobia. In D. H. Barlow (Ed.), *Clinical handbook of psychological disorders: A step-by-step treatment manual* (3rd ed., pp. 1–59). New York: Guilford Press.

Craske, M. G., & Barlow, D. H. (2008). Panic disorder and agoraphobia. In D. H. Barlow (Ed.) *Clinical handbook of psychological disorders: A step-by-step treatment manual* (4th ed., pp. 1–64). New York: Guilford Press.

Dattilio, F. M. (Ed.). (1998). *Case studies in couple and family therapy.* New York: Guilford Press.

Dattilio, F. M. (2005). The restructuring of family schemas: A cognitive-behavior perspective. *Journal of Marital and Family Therapy, 31,* 15–30.

Dattilio, F. M., & Bevilacqua, L. J. (Eds.). (2000). *Comparative treatments for relationship dysfunction.* New York: Springer.

Dattilio, F. M., & Epstein, N. B. (2003). Cognitive-behavior couple and family therapy. In T. L. Sexton, G. R. Weeks, & M. S. Robbins (Eds.), *Handbook of family therapy* (pp. 147–173). New York: Brunner-Routledge.

Davis, S. D. (2005). *Common and model-specific factors: What marital family therapy model developers, their former students, and their clients say about change.* Unpublished doctoral dissertation; Virginia Polytechnic Institute and State University.

Davis, S. D., & Butler, M. H. (2004). Enacting relationships in marriage family therapy: A conceptual and operational definition of an enactment. *Journal of Marital and Family Therapy. 30,* 319–333.

Davis, S. D., & Piercy, F. P. (2007a). What clients of couple therapy model developers and their former students say about change, part I: Model-dependent common factors across three models. *Journal of Marital and Family Therapy, 33,* 318–343.

Davis, S. D., & Piercy, F. P. (2007b). What clients of couple therapy model developers and their former students say about change, part II: Model-independent common factors and an integrative framework. *Journal of Marital and Family Therapy, 33,* 344–363.

deShazer, S. (1985). *Keys to solution in brief therapy.* New York: Norton.

deShazer, S. (1988). *Clues: Investigating solutions in brief therapy.* New York: Norton.

Doherty, W. J., & Beaton, J. M. (2000). Family therapist, community, and civic renewal. *Family Process, 39,* 149–162.

Duncan, B. L., & Miller, S. D. (2000). *The heroic client: Doing client-directed, outcome-informed therapy.* San Francisco: Jossey-Bass.

Duncan, B. L., Miller, S. D., & Sparks, J. A. (2004). *The heroic client: A revolutionary way to improve effectiveness through client-directed, outcome-informed therapy* (rev. ed.). San Francisco: Jossey-Bass.

Duncan, B. L., Sparks, J. A., & Miller, S. D. (2006). Client, not theory, directed: Integrating approaches one client at a time. In G. Stricker & J. Gold (Eds.), *A casebook of psychotherapy integration* (pp. 225–240). Washington, DC: American Psychological Association.

Elkin, I. (1994). The NIMH Treatment of Depression Collaborative Research Program: Where we began and where we are. In A. E. Bergin & S. L. Garfield (Eds.), *Handbook of psychotherapy and behavior change* (4th ed., pp. 114–139). Oxford, England: Wiley.

Elkin, I. (1999). A major dilemma in psychotherapy outcome research: Disentangling therapists from therapies. *Clinical Psychology: Science and Practice, 6*(1), 10–32.

Elkin, I., Shea, T., Watkins, J. T., Imber, S. D., Sotsky, S. M., Collins, J. F., et al. (1989). National Institute of Mental Health treatment of depression collaborative research program: General effectiveness of treatments. *Archives of General Psychiatry, 46,* 971–982.

Elliott, R., Watson, J. C., Goldman, R. N., & Greenberg, L. S. (2004). Adapting process-experiential therapy to particular client problems. In R. Elliott, J. C. Watson, R. N. Goldman, & L. S. Greenberg (Eds.), *Learning emotion-focused therapy: The process-experiential approach to change* (pp. 287–310). Washington, DC: American Psychological Association.

Ellis, A. (1962). *Reason and emotion in psychotherapy.* Oxford, England: Lyle Stuart.

Emmelkamp, P. M. G. (2004). In M. J. Lambert (Ed.), *Bergin and Garfield's handbook of psychotherapy and behavior change* (5th ed., pp. 393–446). New York: Wiley.

Engle, G. L. (1977). The need for a new medical model: A challenge for biomedicine. *Science, 196,* 129–136.

Falicov, C. J. (2003). Culture in family therapy: New variations on a fundamental theme. In T. L. Sexton, G. R. Weeks, & M. S. Robbins (Eds.), *Handbook of family therapy: The science and practice of working with families and couples* (pp. 37–55). New York: Brunner-Routledge.

Falloon, I. R. H. (1993). Behavioral family therapy for schizophrenic and affective disorders. In A. S. Bellack & M. Hersen (Eds.), *Handbook of behavior therapy in the psychiatric setting* (pp. 595–611). New York: Plenum Press.

Falloon, I. R. H. (2002). Cognitive-behavioral family and educational interventions for schizophrenic disorders. In S. G. Hofmann & M. C. Tompson (Eds.), *Treating chronic and severe mental disorders: A handbook of empirically supported interventions.* New York: Guilford Press.

Farber, B. A., & Lane, J. S. (2002). Positive regard. In J. C. Norcross (Ed.),

Psychotherapy relationships that work (pp. 175–194). New York: Oxford University Press.

Fisch, R., Weakland, J. H., & Segal, L. (1983). *The tactics of change.* San Francisco: Jossey-Bass.

Fraenkel, P. (2006). Engaging families as experts: Collaborative family program development. *Family Process, 45,* 237–257.

Frank, J. D. (1961). *Persuasion and healing: A comparative study of psychotherapy.* Baltimore: Johns Hopkins University Press.

Frank, J. D. (1973). *Persuasion and healing: A comparative study of psychotherapy* (2nd ed.). Oxford, England: Schocken.

Frank, J. D. (1976). Psychotherapy and the sense of mastery. In R. L. Spitzer & D. F. Klein (Eds.), *Evaluation of psychotherapies: Behavior therapies, drug therapies, and their interactions* (pp. 47–56). Baltimore: Johns Hopkins University Press.

Frank, J. D., & Frank, J. B. (1991). *Persuasion and healing: A comparative study of psychotherapy* (3rd ed.). Baltimore: Johns Hopkins University Press.

Franklin, M. E., & Foa, E. B. (2007). Cognitive behavioral treatment of obsessive–compulsive disorder. In P. E. Nathan & J. M. Gorman (Eds.), *A guide to treatments that work* (3rd ed., pp. 431–446). New York: Oxford University Press.

Freud, S. (1987). The origin and development of psychoanalysis: First and second lectures. *American Journal of Psychology, 100*(3–4), 472–488.

Friedlander, M. L., Escudero, V., & Heatherington, L. (2006a). Building and maintaining healthy alliances. In *Therapeutic alliances in couple and family therapy: An empirically informed guide to practice* (pp. 261–268). Washington, DC: American Psychological Association.

Friedlander, M. L., Escudero, V., & Heatherington, L. (2006b). Building blocks of the alliance. In *Therapeutic alliances in couple and family therapy: An empirically informed guide to practice* (pp. 143–158). Washington, DC: American Psychological Association.

Friedlander, M. L., Escudero, V., & Heatherington, L. (2006c). *Therapeutic alliances in couple and family therapy: An empirically informed guide to practice.* Washington, DC: American Psychological Association.

Friedlander, M. L., Escudero, V., Horvath, A. O., Heatherington, L., Cabero, A., & Martens, M. P. (2006). System for observing family therapy alliances: A tool for research and practice. *Journal of Counseling Psychology, 53*(2), 214–225.

Furman, B., & Ahola, T. (1994). Solution talk: The solution-oriented way of talking about problems. In M. F. Hoyt (Ed.), *Constructive therapies* (pp. 41–66). New York: Guilford Press.

Garfield, S. L. (1987). Towards a scientifically oriented eclecticism. *Scandinavian Journal of Behavior Therapy, 16,* 95–109.

Goldfried, M. R. (1980). Toward the delineation of therapeutic change principles. *American Psychologist, 35,* 991–995.

Goldfried, M. R., & Norcross, J. C. (1995). Integrative and eclectic therapies in historical perspective. In B. M. Bongar & L. E. Beutler (Eds.), *Comprehensive textbook of psychotherapy: Theory and practice* (pp. 254–273). London: Oxford University Press.

Goldfried, M. R., & Padaver, W. (1982). Current status and future directions in psychotherapy. In M. R. Goldfried (Ed.), *Converging themes in psychotherapy* (pp. 3–49). New York: Springer.

Gottman, J. M. (1994). *Why marriages succeed or fail.* New York: Simon & Schuster.

Gottman, J. M., & Notarious, C. I. (2000). Decade review: Observing marital interaction. *Journal of Marriage and the Family, 62,* 927–947.

Gottman, J. M., & Silver, N. (1999). *The seven principles for making marriage work.* New York: Three Rivers Press.

Green, R.-J., & Herget, M. (1991). Outcomes of systemic/strategic team consultation: III. The importance of therapist warmth and active structuring. *Family Process, 30*(3), 321–336.

Greenberg, L. S., & Pinsof, W. M. (Eds.). (1986). *The psychotherapeutic process: A research handbook.* New York: Guilford Press.

Greenberg, L. S., & Watson, J. (1998). Experiential therapy of depression: Differential effects of client-centered relationship conditions and process experiential interventions. *Psychotherapy Research, 8*(2), 210–224.

Grencavage, L. M., & Norcross, J. C. (1990). Where are the commonalities among the therapeutic common factors? *Professional Psychology Research and Practice, 21,* 372–378.

Gurman, A. S. (1978). Contemporary marital therapies: A critique and comparative analysis of psychoanalytic, behavioral and systems theory approaches. In T. J. Paolino & B. S. McCrady (Eds.), *Marriage and marital therapy: Psychoanalytic, behavioral and systems theory perspectives* (pp. 445–566). Oxford, England: Brunner/Mazel.

Haaga, D. A., McCrady, B., & Lebow, J. (2006). Integrative principles for treating substance use disorders. *Journal of Clinical Psychology, 62*(6), 675–684.

Haas, L. J., Alexander, J. F., & Mas, C. (1988). Functional Family Therapy: Basic concepts and training program. In H. A. Liddle, D. C. Breunlin, & R. C. Schwartz (Eds.), *Handbook of family therapy training and supervision* (pp. 128–147). New York: Guilford Press.

Haley, J. (1987). *Problem-solving therapy* (2nd ed.). San Francisco: Jossey-Bass.

Haley, J. (1997). *Leaving home: The therapy of disturbed young people* (2nd ed.). Philadelphia: Brunner/Mazel.

Harmon, C., Hawkins, E. J., Lambert, M. J., Slade, K., & Whipple, J. S. (2005). Improving outcomes for poorly responding clients: The use of clinical support tools and feedback to clients. *Journal of Clinical Psychology, 61*(2), 175–185.

Heimann, P. (1950). On counter-transference. *International Journal of Psycho-Analysis, 31,* 81–84.

Helmeke, K. B., & Sprenkle, D. H. (2000). Clients' perceptions of pivotal moments in couples therapy: A qualitative study of change in therapy. *Journal of Marital and Family Therapy, 26,* 469–484.

Henggeler, S. W., & Lee, T. (2003). Multisystemic treatment of serious clinical problems. In A. E. Kazdin & J. R. Weisz (Eds.), *Evidence-based psychotherapies for children and adolescents* (pp. 301–322). New York: Guilford Press.

Henggeler, S. W., Schoenwald, S. K., Borduin, C. M., Rowland, M. D., & Cunningham, P. B. (1998). *Multisystemic treatment of antisocial behavior in children and adolescents.* New York: Guilford Press.

Henggeler, S. W., Schoenwald, S. K., Rowland, M. D., & Cunningham, P. B. (2002). *Serious emotional disturbance in children and adolescents: Multisystemic therapy.* New York: Guilford Press.

Henggeler, S. W., & Sheidow, A. J. (2002). Conduct disorder and delinquency. In D. H. Sprenkle (Ed.), *Effectiveness research in marriage and family therapy* (pp. 27–52). Alexandria, VA: American Association for Marriage and Family Therapy.

Hollander-Goldfein, B. (1989). Basic principles: Structural elements of the intersystem approach. In G. R. Weeks (Ed.), *Treating couples: The intersystem model of the Marriage Council of Philadelphia* (pp. 38–69). New York: Brunner Mazel.

Hollon, S. T., & Beck, A. T. (2004). Cognitive and cognitive behavioral therapies. In M. J. Lambert (Ed.), *Bergin and Garfield's handbook of psychotherapy and behavior change* (5th ed., pp. 447–492). New York: Wiley.

Holtzworth-Munroe, A., Jacobson, N. S., DeKlyen, M., & Whisman, M. A. (1989). Relationship between behavioral marital therapy outcome and process variables. *Journal of Consulting and Clinical Psychology, 57,* 658–662.

Horvath, A. O. (Ed.). (1994). *Empirical validation of Bordin's pantheoretical model of the alliance: The Working Alliance Inventory perspective.* Oxford, England: Wiley.

Horvath, A. O. (2001). The alliance. *Psychotherapy: Theory, Research, Practice, Training, 38*(4), 365–372.

Horvath, A. O. (2006). The alliance in context: Accomplishments, challenges, and future directions. *Psychotherapy: Theory, Research, Practice, Training, 43*(3), 258–263.

Horvath, A. O., & Bedi, R. P. (Eds.). (2002). *The alliance.* New York: Oxford University Press.

Horvath, A. O., & Greenberg, L. S. (1989). Development and validation of the Working Alliance Inventory. *Journal of Counseling Psychology, 36*(2), 223–233.

Horvath, A. O., & Greenberg, L. S. (Eds.). (1994). *The working alliance: Theory, research, and practice.* Oxford, England: Wiley.

Howard, K. I., Moras, K., Brill, P. L., Martinovich, Z., & Lutz, W. (1996). The evaluation of psychotherapy: Efficacy, effectiveness, and patient progress. *American Psychologist, 51*, 1059–1064.

Howard, K. I., Orlinsky, D. E., Saunders, S. M., Bankoff, E., Davidson, C., & O'Mahoney, M. T. (1991). Northwestern University–University of Chicago Psychotherapy Research Program. In *Psychotherapy research: An international review of programmatic studies* (pp. 65–74). Washington, DC: American Psychological Association.

Hubble, M. A., Duncan, B. L., & Miller, S. D. (Eds.). (1999). *The heart and soul of change: What works in therapy.* Washington, DC: American Psychological Association.

Jacobson, N. S. (1980). Behavioral marital therapy: Current trends in research, assessment and practice. *American Journal of Family Therapy, 8*(2), 3–5.

Jacobson, N. S., & Christensen, A. (1996). *Integrative couple therapy: Promoting acceptance and change.* New York: Norton.

Jacobson, N. S., Christensen, A., Prince, S. E., Cordova, J., & Eldridge, K. (2000). Integrative behavioral couple therapy: An acceptance-based, promising new treatment for couple discord. *Journal of Consulting and Clinical Psychology, 68*(2), 351–355.

Jacobson, N. S., Dobson, K., Fruzzetti, A. E., Schmaling, K. B., & Salusky, S. (1991). Marital therapy as a treatment for depression. *Journal of Consulting and Clinical Psychology, 59*(4), 547–557.

Johnson, S. M. (1996). *Creating connection: The practice of emotionally focused marital therapy.* New York: Brunner/Mazel.

Johnson, S. M. (2002). Marital problems. In D. H. Sprenkle (Ed.), *Effectiveness research in marriage and family therapy* (pp. 163–190). Alexandria, VA: American Association for Marriage and Family Therapy.

Johnson, S. M. (2003a). Couples therapy research: Status and directions. In G. Sholevar (Ed.), *Textbook of family and couples therapy: Clinical applications* (pp. 797–814). Washington, DC: American Psychiatric Publishing.

Johnson, S. M. (2003b). Emotionally focused couples therapy: Empiricism and art. In T. L. Sexton, G. R. Weeks, & M. S. Robbins (Eds.), *Handbook of family therapy: The science and practice of working with families and couples* (pp. 263–280). New York: Brunner-Routledge.

Johnson, S. M. (2004). *The practice of emotionally focused marital therapy: Creating connection* (2nd ed.). New York: Brunner/Mazel.

Johnson, S. M., & Denton, W. (2002). Emotionally focused couple therapy: Creating secure connections. In A. S. Gurman & N. S. Jacobson (Eds.), *Clinical handbook of couple therapy* (3rd ed., pp. 221–250). New York: Guilford Press.

Johnson, S. M., & Talitman, E. (1997). Predictors of success in Emotionally Focused Marital Therapy. *Journal of Marital and Family Therapy, 23*, 135–152.

Jung, C. (1916). On some crucial points in psychoanalysis. In C. G. Jung & C. E. Long (Eds.), *Analytical psychology* (pp. 236–277). New York: Moffat & Yard.

Jung, C. (1935). Basic principles of practical psychotherapy. *Zentralblatt für Psychotherapie, 8,* 66–82.

Karasu, T. B. (1986). The specificity versus nonspecificity dilemma: Toward identifying therapeutic change agents. *American Journal of Psychiatry, 143,* 687–695.

Kazantzis, N., & L'Abate, L. (2007). *Handbook of homework assignments in psychotherapy: Research, practice, prevention.* New York: Springer.

Kazdin, A. E. (Ed.). (2003). *Methodological issues and strategies in clinical research* (3rd ed.). Washington, DC: American Psychological Association.

Kazdin, A. E. (2007). Psychosocial treatments for conduct disorder in children and adolescents. In P. E. Nathan & J. M. Gorman (Eds.), *A guide to treatments that work* (3rd ed., pp. 71–104). New York: Oxford University Press.

Keith, D. V., Connell, G. M., & Whitaker, C. A. (1991). A symbolic–experiential approach to the resolution of therapeutic obstacles in family therapy. *Journal of Family Psychotherapy, 2*(3), 41–56.

Kerr, M. E., & Bowen, M. (1988). *Family evaluation: An approach to Bowen theory.* New York: Norton.

Kiser, D. J., Piercy, F. P., & Lipchik, E. (1993). The integration of emotion in solution-focused therapy. *Journal of Marital and Family Therapy, 19,* 233–242.

Klerman, G. L., & Weissman, M. M. (1991). Interpersonal psychotherapy: Research program and future prospects. In L. E. Beutler & M. Crago (Eds.), *Psychotherapy research: An international review of programmatic studies* (pp. 33–40). Washington, DC: American Psychological Association.

Klerman, G. L., Weissman, M. M., Rounsaville, B., & Chevron, E. S. (1995). Interpersonal psychotherapy for depression. *Journal of Psychotherapy Practice and Research, 4*(4), 342–351.

Knobloch-Fedders, L. M., Pinsof, W. M., & Mann, B. J. (2004). The formation of the therapeutic alliance in couple therapy. *Family Process, 43*(4), 425–442.

Knobloch-Fedders, L. M., Pinsof, W. M., & Mann, B. J. (2007). Therapeutic alliance and treatment progress in couple psychotherapy. *Journal of Marital and Family Therapy, 33*(2), 245–257.

Koerner, K., & Linehan, M. M. (2002). Dialectical behavior therapy for borderline personality disorder. In S. G. Hofmann & M. C. Tompson (Eds.), *Treating chronic and severe mental disorders: A handbook of empirically supported interventions* (pp. 317–342). New York: Guilford Press.

Kolden, G. G., & Howard, K. I. (1992). An empirical test of the generic model of psychotherapy. *Journal of Psychotherapy Practice and Research, 1*(3), 225–236.

Krupnick, J. L., Elkin, I., Collins, J., Simmens, S., Sotsby, S., Pilkonis, P., et al. (1994). Therapeutic alliance and clinical outcome in the NIMH Treatment of Depression Collaborative Research Program: Preliminary findings. *Psychotherapy: Theory, Research, Practice, Training, 31*(1), 28–35.

Kuehl, B. P., Newfield, N. A., & Joanning, H. (1990). A client-based description of family therapy. *Journal of Family Psychology, 3,* 310–321.

Lambert, M. J. (1992). Psychotherapy outcome research: Implications for integrative and eclectic therapists. In J. C. Norcross & M. R. Goldfried (Eds.), *Handbook of psychotherapy integration* (pp. 94–129). New York: Basic Books.

Lambert, M. J. (Ed.). (2004). *Bergin and Garfield's handbook of psychotherapy and behavior change* (5th ed.). New York: Wiley.

Lambert, M. J. (2005). Early response in psychotherapy: Further evidence for the importance of common factors rather than "placebo effects." *Journal of Clinical Psychology, 61*(7), 855–869.

Lambert, M. J., & Bergin, A. E. (1994). The effectiveness of psychotherapy. In A. E. Bergin & S. L. Garfield (Eds.), *Handbook of psychotherapy and behavior change* (4th ed., pp. 143–189). Oxford, England: Wiley.

Lambert, M. J., Harmon, C., Slade, K., Whipple, J. L., & Hawkins, E. J. (2005). Providing feedback to psychotherapists on their patients' progress: Clinical results and practice suggestions. *Journal of Clinical Psychology, 61(2),* 165–174.

Lambert, M. J., & Hill, C. E. (1994). Assessing psychotherapy outcomes and processes. In A. E. Bergin & S. L. Garfield (Eds.), *Handbook of psychotherapy and behavior change* (4th ed., pp. 72–113). Oxford, England: Wiley.

Lambert, M. J., & Ogles, B. M. (2004). The efficacy and effectiveness of psychotherapy. In M. J. Lambert (Ed.), *Bergin and Garfield's handbook of psychotherapy and behavior change* (5th ed., pp. 139–193). New York: Wiley.

Lebow, J. L. (1982). Consumer satisfaction with mental health treatment. *Psychological Bulletin, 91*(2), 244–259.

Lebow, J. L. (1987). Developing a personal integration in family therapy: Principles for model construction and practice. *Journal of Marital and Family Therapy, 13*(1), 1–14.

Lebow, J. L. (1995). Open-ended therapy: Termination in marital and family therapy. In *Integrating family therapy: Handbook of family psychology and systems theory* (pp. 73–86). Washington, DC: American Psychological Association.

Lebow, J. L. (1997). The integrative revolution in couple and family therapy. *Family Process, 36*(1), 1–17.

Lebow, J. L. (2002). Training in integrative/eclectic psychotherapy. In F. W.

Kaslow (Ed.), *Comprehensive handbook of psychotherapy: Vol. 4. Integrative/eclectic* (pp. 545–556). Hoboken, NJ: Wiley.

Lebow, J. L. (2005). Integrative family therapy for families experiencing high-conflict divorce. In J. L. Lebow (Ed.), *Handbook of clinical family therapy* (pp. 516–542). Hoboken, NJ: Wiley.

Lebow, J. L. (2006a). Integrative couple therapy. In G. Stricker & J. Gold (Eds.), *A casebook of psychotherapy integration* (pp. 211–223). Washington, DC: American Psychological Association.

Lebow, J. L. (2006b). *Research for the psychotherapist: From science to practice*. New York: Routledge.

Lebow, J. L. (2008). *Twenty-first century psychotherapies: Contemporary approaches to theory and practice*. Hoboken, NJ: Wiley.

Leon, S. C., Kopta, S., Howard, K. I., & Lutz, W. (1999). Predicting patients' responses to psychotherapy: Are some more predictable than others? *Journal of Consulting and Clinical Psychology, 67*(5), 698–704.

Liddle, H. A., Rodriguez, R. A., Dakof, G. A., Kanzki, E., & Marvel, F. A. (2005). Multidimensional family therapy: A science-based treatment for adolescent drug abuse. In J. L. Lebow (Ed.), *Handbook of clinical family therapy* (pp. 128–163). Hoboken, NJ: Wiley.

Liddle, H. A., & Rowe, C. L. (2002). Multidimensional family therapy for adolescent drug abuse: Making the case for a developmental–contextual, family-based intervention. In D. W. Brook & H. I. Spitz (Eds.), *The group therapy of substance abuse* (pp. 275–291). New York: Haworth Press.

Liddle, H. A., Rowe, C. L., Quille, T. J., Dakof, G. A., Mills, D. S., Sakran, E., et al. (2002). Transporting a research-based adolescent drug treatment into practice. *Journal of Substance Abuse Treatment, 22*, 231–243.

Linehan, M. M., Schmidt, H., III, Dimeff, L. A., Craft, J., Kanter, J., & Comtois, K. A. (1999). Dialectical behavior therapy for patients with borderline personality disorder and drug-dependence. *American Journal on Addictions, 8*(4), 279–292.

Lipchik, E. (1988). Purposeful sequences for beginning the solution-focused interview. *Family Therapy Collections, 24*, 105–117.

Luborsky, L., Crits-Christoph, P., McLellan, A. T., Woody, G., Piper, W., Liberman, B., et al. (1986). Do therapists vary much in their success?: Findings from four outcome studies. *American Journal of Orthopsychiatry, 56*, 501–512.

Luborsky, L., Diguer, L., Seligman, D. A., Rosenthal, R., Johnson, S. Halperin, G., et al. (1999). The researcher's own therapeutic alliances: A "wild card" in comparisons of treatment efficacy. *Clinical Psychology: Science and Practice. 6*, 95–132.

Luborsky, L., Rosenthal, R., Diguer, L., Andrusyna, T. P., Berman, J. S., Levitt, J. T., et al. (2002). The dodo bird verdict is alive and well—mostly. *Clinical Psychology: Science and Practice, 9*, 2–12.

Luborsky, L., Singer, B., & Luborsky, L. (1975). Comparative studies of psychotherapy: Is it true that "Everyone has won and all must have prizes"? *Archives of General Psychiatry, 32,* 995–1008.

Markman, H. J., Stanley, S. M., & Blumberg, S. L. (1996). *Fighting for your marriage: Positive steps for preventing divorce and preserving a lasting love* (2nd ed.). San Francisco: Jossey-Bass.

Maturana, H. R. (1992). *Biology, emotions and culture* [Videotape 6]. Calgary, Canada: Vanry & Associates.

McCarthy, B. W. (2002). Sexuality, sexual dysfunction, and couple therapy. In A. S. Gurman & N. S. Jacobson (Eds.), *Clinical handbook of couple therapy* (3rd ed., pp. 629–652). New York: Guilford Press.

McFarlane, W. R., Dixon, L., & Lucksted, A. (2002). Severe mental illness. In D. H. Sprenkle (Ed.), *Effectiveness research in marriage and family therapy* (pp. 255–288). Alexandria, VA: American Association for Marriage and Family Therapy.

McGoldrick, M., Giordano, J., & Garcia-Preto, N. (Eds.). (2005). *Ethnicity and family therapy* (3rd ed.). New York: Guilford Press.

McGoldrick, M., Giordano, J., & Pearce, J. K. (Eds.). (1996). *Ethnicity and family therapy* (2nd ed.). New York: Guilford Press.

Middleberg, C. V. (2001). Projective identification in common couples dances. *Journal of Marital and Family Therapy, 27,* 341–352.

Miklowitz, D. J. (2008). *Bipolar disorder: A family-focused treatment approach* (2nd ed.). New York: Guilford Press.

Miklowitz, D. J., Richards, J. A., George, E. L., Frank, E., Suddath, R. L., Powell, K. B., et al. (2003). Integrated family and individual therapy for bipolar disorder: Results of a treatment development study. *Journal of Clinical Psychiatry, 64*(2), 182–191.

Miklowitz, D. J., Simoneau, T. L., George, E. L., Richards, J. A., Kalbag, A., Sachs-Ericsson, N., et al. (2000). Family-focused treatment of bipolar disorder: 1-year effects of a psychoeducational program in conjunction with pharmacotherapy. *Biological Psychiatry, 48*(6), 582–592.

Miller, G., & deShazer, S. (2000). Emotions in solution-focused therapy: A re-examination. *Family Process, 39,* 5–23.

Miller, S. D., Duncan, B. L., & Hubble, M. A. (1997). *Escape from Babel: Toward a unifying language for psychotherapy practice.* New York: Norton.

Miller, S. D., Duncan, B. L., & Hubble, M. A. (2005). Outcome-informed clinical work. In J. C. Norcross & M. R. Goldfried (Eds.), *Handbook of psychotherapy integration* (2nd ed., pp. 84–102). London: Oxford University Press.

Miller, S. D., Duncan, B. L., Sorrell, R., & Brown, G. S. (2005). The Partners Behavior Change Outcome Management System. *Journal of Clinical Psychology, 61*(2), 199–208.

Miller, S. D., Hubble, M., & Duncan, B. (2007, November–December). Supershrinks. *Psychotherapy Networker,* pp. 26–35, 56.

Miller, W. R. (1995). *Motivational enhancement therapy with drug abus-*

ers. Treatment manual funded by the National Institute on Drug Abuse (RO1-DA08896).

Miller, W. R. (2000). Motivational interviewing IV: Some parallels with horse whispering. *Behavioural and Cognitive Psychotherapy, 28,* 285–292.

Miller, W. R., & Rollnick, S. (2002). *Motivational interviewing: Preparing people for change* (2nd ed.). New York: Guilford Press.

Miller, W. R., & Rollnick, S. (2003). Motivational interviewing: Preparing people for change. *American Journal of Forensic Psychology, 21*(1), 83–85.

Minuchin, S. (1974). *Families and family therapy.* Cambridge, MA: Harvard University Press.

Minuchin, S. (1998). Where is the family in narrative family therapy? *Journal of Marital and Family Therapy, 24,* 397–404.

Minuchin, S., & Fishman, H. C. (1981). *Family therapy techniques.* Cambridge, MA: Harvard University Press.

Mitrani, V. B., Prado, G., Feaster, D. J., Robinson-Batista, C., & Szapocznik, J. (2003). Relational factors and family treatment engagement among low-income, HIV-positive African American mothers. *Family Process, 42*(1), 31–45.

Muir, J. A., Schwartz, S. J., & Szapocznik, J. (2004). A program of research with Hispanic and African American families: Three decades of intervention development and testing influenced by the changing cultural context of Miami. *Journal of Marital and Family Therapy, 30,* 113–129.

Murphy, C. M., & Eckhardt, C. I. (2005). *Treating the abusive partner: An individualized cognitive-behavioral approach.* New York: Guilford Press.

Napier, A. (1997, September). *Called by families: The journey of the therapist.* Plenary address at the annual meeting of the American Association for Marriage and Family Therapy, Atlanta, GA.

Nichols, M. P., & Schwartz, R. C. (2001). *Family therapy: Concepts and methods* (5th ed.). Boston: Allyn & Bacon.

Norcross, J. C. (2002a). Empirically supported therapy relationships. In J. C. Norcross (Ed.), *Psychotherapy relationships that work: Therapist contributions and responsiveness to patients* (pp. 3–16). London: Oxford University Press.

Norcross, J. C. (Ed.). (2002b). *Psychotherapy relationships that work: Therapist contributions and responsiveness to patients.* London: Oxford University Press.

Norcross, J. C., & Newman, C. F. (1992). Psychotherapy integration: Setting the context. In J. C. Norcross & M. R. Goldfried (Eds.), *Handbook of psychotherapy integration* (pp. 3–45). New York: Basic Books.

O'Farrell, T. J., & Fals-Stewart, W. F. (2002). Alcohol abuse. In D. H. Sprenkle (Ed.), *Effectiveness research in marriage and family therapy* (pp. 123–161). Alexandria, VA: American Association for Marriage and Family Therapy.

O'Hanlon, W. H., & Beadle, S. (1997). *A guide to possibility land: Fifty-one methods for doing brief, respectful therapy.* New York: Norton.

Onedera, J. D. (2006). Functional family therapy: An interview with Dr. James Alexander. *The Family Journal, 14,* 306–311.

Orlinsky, D. E., Grawe, K., & Parks, B. K. (1994). Process and outcome in psychotherapy: Nocheinmal. In A. E. Bergin & S. L. Garfield (Eds.), *Handbook of psychotherapy and behavior change* (4th ed., pp. 270–376). Oxford, England: Wiley.

Orlinsky, D. E., & Howard, K. I. (1987). A generic model of psychotherapy. *Journal of Integrative and Eclectic Psychotherapy, 6*(1), 6–27.

Orlinsky, D. E., & Ronnestad, M. (2000). Ironies in the history of psychotherapy research: Rogers, Bordin, and the shape of things that came. *Journal of Clinical Psychology, 56*(7), 841–851.

Patterson, C. H. (1984). Empathy, warmth, and genuineness in psychotherapy: A review of reviews. *Psychotherapy: Theory, Research, Practice, Training, 21,* 431–438.

Peterson, C., & Seligman, M. E. (2004). Social Intelligence. In C. Peterson & M. E. Seligman (Eds.), *Character strengths and virtues: A handbook and classification* (pp. 337–353). Washington, DC: American Psychological Association.

Pickrel, S. G., & Henggeler, S. W. (1996). Multisystemic therapy for adolescent substance abuse and dependence. *Child and Adolescent Psychiatric Clinics of North America, 5*(1), 201–211.

Piercy, F. P., Lipchik, E., & Kiser, D. (2000). Miller and DeShazer's article on "emotions in solution-focused therapy." *Family Process, 39,* 25–28.

Pinsof, W. M. (1978). *Family therapist verbal behavior: Development of a coding system.* Toronto, Canada: York University.

Pinsof, W. M. (1995). *Integrative problem-centered therapy: A synthesis of family, individual, and biological therapies.* New York: Basic Books.

Pinsof, W. M. (2005). Integrative problem-centered therapy. In J. C. Norcross & M. R. Goldfried (Eds.), *Handbook of psychotherapy integration* (2nd ed., pp. 382–402). New York: Oxford University Press.

Pinsof, W. M., & Catherall, D. R. (1986). The integrative psychotherapy alliance: Family, couple and individual therapy scales. *Journal of Marital and Family Therapy, 12*(2), 137–151.

Pinsof, W. M., & Lebow, J. L. (2005). A scientific paradigm for family psychology. In W. M. Pinsof & J. L. Lebow (Eds.), *Family psychology: The art of the science* (pp. 3–19). New York: Oxford University Press.

Pinsof, W. M., & Wynne, L. C. (Eds.). (1995). *Family therapy effectiveness: Current research and theory.* Alexandria, VA: American Association for Marriage and Family Therapy.

Pinsof, W. M., Zinbarg, R., & Knobloch-Fedders, L. M. (2008). Factoria and construct validity of the revised short form Integrative Psychotherapy Alliance Scales for Family, Couple, and Individual Psychotherapy. *Family Process, 47,* 281–301.

Prochaska, J. O. (1994). Strong and weak principles for progressing from precontemplation to action on the basis of twelve problem behaviors. *Health Psychology, 13,* 47–51.

Prochaska, J. O. (1999). How do people change, and how can we change to help many more people? In M. A. Hubble, B. L. Duncan, & S. D. Miller (Eds.), *The heart and soul of change* (pp. 227–255). Washington, DC: American Psychological Association.

Prochaska, J. O., DiClemente, C. C., & Norcross, J. C. (1992). In search of how people change: Applications to addictive behaviors. *American Psychologist, 47,* 1102–1114.

Prochaska, J. O., Velicer, W. F., & Rossi, J. S. (1994). Stages of change and decisional balance for 12 problem behaviors. *Health Psychology, 13,* 39–46.

Project MATCH Research Group. (1997). Matching alcoholism treatments to client heterogeneity: Project MATCH posttreatment drinking outcomes. *Journal of Studies in Alcoholism, 58,* 7–29.

Raskin, N. J., & Rogers, C. R. (1989). Person-centered therapy. In R. J. Corsini & D. Wedding (Eds.), *Current psychotherapies* (4th ed., pp. 155–194). Itasca, IL: Peacock.

Rea, M. M., Tompson, M. C., Miklowitz, D. J., Goldstein, M. J., Hwang, S., & Mintz, J. (2003). Family-focused treatment versus individual treatment for bipolar disorder: Results of a randomized clinical trial. *Journal of Consulting and Clinical Psychology, 71*(3), 482–492.

Robbins, M. S., Alexander, J. F., Newell, R. M., & Turner, C. W. (1996). The immediate effect of reframing on client attitude in family therapy. *Journal of Family Psychology, 10*(1), 28–34.

Robbins, M. S., Szapocznik, J., Santisteban, D. A., Hervis, O. E., Mitrani, V. B., & Schwartz, S. J. (2003). Brief strategic family therapy for Hispanic youth. In A. E. Kazdin & J. R. Weisz (Eds.), *Evidence-based psychotherapies for children and adolescents* (pp. 407–424). New York: Guilford Press.

Rogers, C. R. (1951). The necessary and sufficient conditions of therapeutic personality change. *Journal of Consulting Psychology, 21,* 95–103.

Rogers, C. R. (1961). *On becoming a person.* London: Constable.

Rogers, C. R., Kirschenbaum, H., & Henderson, V. L. (1989). *The Carl Rogers reader.* Boston: Houghton Mifflin.

Rosenzweig, S. (1936). Some implicit common factors in diverse methods in psychotherapy. *Journal of Orthopsychiatry, 6,* 412–415.

Rowe, C. L., & Liddle, H. A. (2002). Substance abuse. In D. H. Sprenkle (Ed.), *Effectiveness research in marriage and family therapy* (pp. 53–87). Alexandria, VA: American Association for Marriage and Family Therapy.

Santisteban, D. A., Coatsworth, J., Perez-Vidal, A., Kurtines, W. M., Schwartz, S. J., LaPerriere, A., et al. (2003). Efficacy of brief strategic family therapy in modifying Hispanic adolescent behavior problems and substance use. *Journal of Family Psychology, 17*(1), 121–133.

Santisteban, D. A., & Szapocznik, J. (1994). Bridging theory, research and practice to more successfully engage substance abusing youth and their families into therapy. *Journal of Child and Adolescent Substance Abuse, 3*(2), 9–24.

Santisteban, D. A., Szapocznik, J., Perez-Vidal, A., Kurtines, W. M., Murray, E. J., & LaPerriere, A. (1996). Efficacy of intervention for engaging youth and families into treatment and some variables that may contribute to differential effectiveness. *Journal of Family Psychology, 10*(1), 35–44.

Scharff, D., & Scharff, J. S. (1987). *Object relations family therapy.* New York: Jason Aronson.

Scharff, J. S., & Bagnini, C. (2002). Object relations couple therapy. In A. S. Gurman & N. S. Jacobson (Eds.), *Clinical handbook of couple therapy* (pp. 59–85). New York: Guilford Press.

Sexton, T. L., & Alexander, J. F. (2003). Functional family therapy: A mature clinical model for working with at-risk adolescents and their families. In T. L. Sexton, G. R. Weeks, & M. S. Robbins (Eds.), *Handbook of family therapy: The science and practice of working with families and couples* (pp. 323–348). New York: Brunner-Routledge.

Sexton, T. L., & Alexander, J. F. (2005). Functional family therapy for externalizing disorders in adolescents. In J. L. Lebow (Ed.) *Handbook of clinical family therapy* (pp. 164–191). Hoboken, NJ: Wiley.

Sexton, T. L., Gilman, L., & Johnson-Erickson, C. (2005). Evidence-based practices. In T. P. Gullota & G. R. Adams (Eds.), *Handbook of adolescent behavioral problems: Evidence-based approaches to prevention and treatment* (pp. 101–128). New York: Springer Science + Business Media.

Sexton, T. L., & Griffin, B. L. (Eds.). (1997). *Constructivist thinking in counseling practice, research, and training.* New York: Teachers College Press.

Sexton, T. L., & Ridley, C. R. (2004). Implications of a moderated common factors approach: Does it move the field forward? *Journal of Marital and Family Therapy, 30*(2), 159–163.

Sexton, T. L., Ridley, C. R., & Kleiner, A. J. (2004). Beyond common factors: Multilevel-process models of therapeutic change in marriage and family therapy. *Journal of Marital & Family Therapy, 30*(2), 131–149.

Shadish, W. R., & Baldwin, S. A. (2002). Meta-analysis of MFT interventions. In D. H. Sprenkle (Ed.), *Effectiveness research in marriage and family therapy* (pp. 339–370). Alexandria, VA: American Association for Marriage and Family Therapy.

Shadish, W. R., & Baldwin, S. A. (2003). Meta-analysis of MFT interventions. *Journal of Marital and Family Therapy, 29*(4), 547–570.

Shadish, W. R., Montgomery, L. M., Wilson, P., Wilson, M. R., Bright, I., &

Okwumabua, T. (1993). Effects of family and marital psychotherapies: A meta-analysis. *Journal of Consulting and Clinical Psychology, 61*(6), 992–1002.

Shadish, W. R., Ragsdale, K., Glaser, R. R., & Montgomery, L. M. (1995). The efficacy and effectiveness of marital and family therapy: A perspective from meta-analysis. *Journal of Marital and Family Therapy, 21*(4), 345–360.

Sheidow, A. J., Henggeler, S. W., Schoenwald, S. K. (2003). Multisystemic therapy. In T. L. Sexton, G. R. Weeks, & M. S. Robbins (Eds.), *Handbook of family therapy* (pp. 323–348). New York: Brunner-Routledge.

Simon, G. M. (2006). The heart of the matter: A proposal for placing the self of the therapist at the center of family therapy research and training. *Family Process, 45*, 331–344.

Smith, M. L., & Glass, G. V. (1977). Meta-analysis of psychotherapy outcome studies. *American Psychologist, 32*(9), 752–760.

Smith, M. L., & Glass, G. V. (1979). Meta-analysis of psychotherapy outcome studies. In C. A. Kiesler, N. A. Cummings, & G. R. VandenBos (Eds.), *Psychology and national health insurance: A sourcebook* (pp. 530–539). Washington, DC: American Psychological Association.

Snow, M. G., Prochaska, J. O., & Rossi, J. S. (1992). Stages of change for smoking cessation among former problem drinkers: A cross-sectional analysis. *Journal of Substance Abuse, 4*, 107–116.

Sprenkle, D. H. (Ed.). (2002). *Effectiveness research in marriage and family therapy*. Alexandria, VA: American Association for Marriage and Family Therapy.

Sprenkle, D. H., & Blow, A. J. (2004a). Common factors and our sacred models. *Journal of Marital and Family Therapy, 30*(2), 113–129.

Sprenkle, D. H., & Blow, A. J. (2004b). Common factors are not islands—they work through models: A response to Sexton, Ridley, and Kleiner. *Journal of Marital and Family Therapy, 30*(2), 151–158.

Sprenkle, D. H., Blow, A. J., & Dickey, M. H. (1999). Common factors and other nontechnique variables in marriage and family therapy. In M. A. Hubble, B. L. Duncan, & S. D. Miller (Eds.), *The heart and soul of change: What works in therapy* (pp. 329–360). Washington, DC: American Psychological Association.

Stith, S. M., Rosen, K. N., & McCollum, E. E. (2002). Domestic violence. In D. H. Sprenkle (Ed.), *Effectiveness research in marriage and family therapy* (pp. 223–254). Alexandria, VA: American Association for Marriage and Family Therapy.

Stolk, Y., & Perlesz, A. J. (1990). Do better trainees make worse family therapists? A follow-up study of client families. *Family Process, 29*, 45–58.

Straus, M. A. (1973). A general systems theory approach to a theory of violence between family members. *Social Science Information, 2*(3), 105–125.

Stricker, G., & Gold, J. (2005). Assimilative Psychodynamic Psychotherapy.

In J. C. Norcross & M. R. Goldfried (Eds.), *Handbook of psychother-apy integration* (2nd ed., pp. 221–240). New York: Oxford University Press.

Szapocznik, J., Kurtines, W. M., Foote, F. H., Perez-Vidal, A., & Hervis, O. (1983). Conjoint versus one-person family therapy: Some evidence for the effectiveness of conducting family therapy through one person. *Journal of Consulting and Clinical Psychology, 51,* 881–899.

Szapocznik, J., Kurtines, W. M., Foote, F. H., Perez-Vidal, A., & Hervis, O. (1986). Conjoint versus one-person family therapy: Further evidence for the effectiveness of conducting family therapy through one person family therapy with drug-abusing adolescents. *Journal of Consulting and Clinical Psychology, 54,* 395–397.

Szapocznik, J., Perez-Vidal, A., Brickman, A. L., Foote, F. H., Santisteban, D., Hervis, O., et al. (1988). Engaging adolescent drug abusers and their families in treatment: A strategic structural systems approach. *Journal of Consulting and Clinical Psychology, 56*(4), 552–557.

Szapocznik, J., Robbins, M. S., Mitrani, V. B., Santisteban, D. A., Hervis, O., & Williams, R. A. (2002). Brief strategic family therapy. In F. W. Kaslow (Ed.), *Comprehensive handbook of psychotherapy: Vol. 4. Integrative/eclectic* (pp. 83–109). New York: Wiley.

Szapocznik, J., & Williams, R. A. (2000). Brief strategic family therapy: Twenty-five years of interplay among theory, research, and practice in adolescent behavior problems and drug abuse. *Clinical Child and Family Psychology Review, 3*(2), 117–134.

Tallman, K., & Bohart, A. C. (1999). The client as a common factor: Clients as self-healers. In M. A. Hubble, B. L. Duncan, & S. D. Miller (Eds.), *The heart and soul of change* (pp. 91–131). Washington, DC: American Psychological Association.

Timm, T. M., & Blow, A. J. (1999). Self-of-therapist work: A balance between removing restraints and identifying resources. *Contemporary Family Therapy: An International Journal, 21,* 331–351.

Waldron, H. B., Turner, C. W., Barton, C., Alexander, J. F., & Cline, V. B. (1997). Therapist defensiveness and marital therapy process and outcome. *American Journal of Family Therapy, 25,* 233–243.

Wampler, K. (1997). *Systems theory and outpatient mental health treatment.* Paper presented at the Inaugural American Association for Marriage and Family Therapy Research Conference, Santa Fe, NM.

Wampold, B. E. (2001). *The great psychotherapy debate: Models, methods, and findings.* Mahwah, NJ: Erlbaum.

Wampold, B. E., Minami, T., Tierney, S. C., Baskin, T. W., & Bhati, K. S. (2005). The placebo is powerful: Estimating placebo effects in medicine and psychotherapy from randomized clinical trials. *Journal of Clinical Psychology, 61*(7), 835–854.

Wampold, B. E., Mondin, G. W., Moody, M., Stich, F., Benson, K., & Ahn, H. (1997). A meta-analysis of outcome studies comparing bona fide psychotherapies: Empiricially, "all must have prizes." *Psychological Bulletin, 122*(3), 203–215.

Wampold, B. E., Ollendick, T. H., & King, N. J. (2006). Do therapies designated as empirically supported treatments for specific disorders produce outcomes superior to non-empirically supported treatment therapies? In J. C. Norcross, L. E. Beutler, & R. F. Levant (Eds.), *Evidence-based practices in mental health: Debate and dialogue on the fundamental questions* (pp. 299–328). Washington, DC: American Psychological Association.

Watzlawick, P., Beavin, J. H., & Jackson, D. (1967). *Pragmatics of human communication: A study of interactional patterns, pathologies, and paradoxes.* New York: Norton.

Watzlawick, P., Weakland, J. H., & Fisch, R. (1974). *Change: Principles of problem formation and problem resolution.* Oxford, England: Norton.

Westen, D., Novotny, C. M., & Thompson-Brenner, H. (2004). The empirical status of empirically supported psychotherapies: Assumptions, findings, and reporting in controlled clinical trials. *Psychological Bulletin, 130,* 631–663.

Westen, D., Stirman, S. W., & DeRubeis, R. J. (2006). Are research patients and clinical trials representative of clinical practice? In J. C. Norcross, L. E. Beutler, & R. F. Levant (Eds.), *Evidence-based practices in mental health: Debate and dialogue on the fundamental questions* (pp. 161–189). Washington, DC: American Psychological Association.

Whitaker, C. A., & Keith, D. M. (1982). Symbolic–experiential family therapy. *Terapia Familiare, 11,* 95–134.

Whitaker, C. A., & Malone, T. P. (1953). *The roots of psychotherapy.* Oxford, England: Blakiston.

White, M., & Epston, D. (1990). *Narrative means to therapeutic ends.* New York: Norton.

Index

219